Engineering Desire

Why do technological promises remain so compelling? Artificial intelligence, digital platforms and algorithmic systems continue to attract extraordinary levels of attention, investment and hope. Their transformative promise persists despite visible shortcomings, recurring disappointments and mounting social and environmental concerns.

Drawing on Lacanian psychoanalysis, Ciano Aydin offers a new way of understanding this enduring appeal. Shifting attention from behavior to desire and from power to receptivity, he reveals the existential dimensions of our investment in algorithmic environments. Using Tinder as a paradigmatic case, the book shows how these environments increasingly organize desire itself by offering recognition, orientation, certainty and the fantasy of wholeness.

But algorithmic environments are not merely sites of illusion. The same systems that sustain fantasies of self-knowledge and completion can also lay bare the structure of desire itself. *Engineering Desire* offers a distinctive framework for understanding both the risks and possibilities of contemporary technological life, rethinking singular self-formation as a possibility within technological mediation.

Ciano Aydin is Full Professor of Philosophy of Technology at the University of Twente, The Netherlands. He is the author of *Extimate Technology: Self-Formation in a Technological World* (Routledge, 2021). He has published in *Transactions of the Charles S. Peirce Society, Phenomenology and the Cognitive Sciences, Journal of Medicine and Philosophy, Philosophy and Technology, AI & Society, Philosophical Psychology* and other journals.

Routledge Focus on Philosophy

Routledge Focus on Philosophy is an exciting and innovative new series, capturing and disseminating some of the best and most exciting new research in philosophy in short book form. Peer reviewed and at a maximum of fifty thousand words shorter than the typical research monograph, *Routledge Focus on Philosophy* titles are available in both ebook and print on demand format. Tackling big topics in a digestible format the series opens up important philosophical research for a wider audience, and as such is invaluable reading for the scholar, researcher and student seeking to keep their finger on the pulse of the discipline. The series also reflects the growing interdisciplinarity within philosophy and will be of interest to those in related disciplines across the humanities and social sciences.

Performative Beauty
A Pragmatist and Somaesthetic Account
Falk Heinrich

The Moral Problems of Competition
Yvette Drissen

War, Pacifism, and Deterrence
A Pragmatist-Transcendental Perspective
Sami Pihlström

Engineering Desire
Algorithmic Environments and the Promise of Wholeness
Ciano Aydin

For more information about this series, please visit: www.routledge.com/Routledge-Focus-on-Philosophy/book-series/RFP

Engineering Desire

Algorithmic Environments and the Promise of Wholeness

Ciano Aydin

Routledge
Taylor & Francis Group
NEW YORK AND LONDON

First published 2027
by Routledge
605 Third Avenue, New York, NY 10158

and by Routledge
4 Park Square, Milton Park, Abingdon, Oxon, OX14 4RN

Routledge is an imprint of the Taylor & Francis Group, an informa business

ISBN: 978-1-041-38002-3 (hbk)
ISBN: 978-1-041-38001-6 (pbk)
ISBN: 978-1-042-01091-2 (ebk)

DOI: 10.4324/9781042010912

Typeset in Times New Roman
by SPi Technologies India Pvt Ltd (Straive)

Contents

Acknowledgments

This book began with a seemingly simple question: Why are we so susceptible to technological promises? Once it appeared, it kept returning, shaping how I thought about technology and the desires bound up with it. It became increasingly clear that it is not enough to study how technologies are built or how they influence and steer behavior. We also need to understand the deeper desire that makes us want to believe in these promises. This book follows that intuition.

The author gratefully acknowledges the financial support provided by the BMS Open Access Fund of the Faculty of BMS at the University of Twente, as well as the ESDIT (Ethics of Socially Disruptive Technologies) project, which supported the open access publication of this book.

Many of the ideas in this book emerged through ongoing conversations with my PhD students, colleagues and friends. Their questions, reflections and critical engagement helped sharpen the arguments and expand the scope of the project. I cannot name them all individually, but they know who they are, and I am deeply grateful to each of them. The theme of desire also has a personal source: an impossible desire rooted in the early loss of my mother. I dedicate this book to her, my object-cause of desire.

1 Introduction

The Economist published a striking headline: "What happened to the artificial-intelligence revolution? So far the technology has had almost no economic impact" (*The Economist*, July 2, 2024). This is remarkable given that the five dominant tech companies, Alphabet, Amazon, Apple, Meta and Microsoft, have collectively invested an estimated $400 billion in AI and related infrastructure and research in that same period. While certain applications these companies offer are emerging and already generating revenue, much of the economic momentum surrounding AI is driven less by what these systems currently achieve and more by expectations regarding what they may eventually become capable of delivering. The resulting valuations and investments are therefore strongly oriented toward projected futures rather than demonstrable present impact.

What AI is ultimately expected to deliver, however, remains remarkably indeterminate. It is not promoted as a solution to a specific, well-defined problem but as a general-purpose, transformative force, a cure-all for every sector, spanning commerce, business, education, public policy, engineering and science. Sometimes this vagueness is addressed by suggesting that we are not building a single AI but a constellation of mutually reinforcing AI technologies and applications that will fundamentally reshape society. Yet this does little to specify what this transformation ultimately consists in. Rather than clarifying the promise, it expands and diffuses it across an ever broader technological horizon. In this way, AI is once again framed not as a tool for solving distinct, concrete problems but as a redemptive promise of boundless applicability.

Meanwhile, AI's limitations are increasingly difficult to ignore (see also Beerends et al. 2026). Across academic and public debates, growing attention has been directed toward the gap between the expansive promises surrounding AI and the actual capacities of current computational systems (Westerstrand et al. 2024; Markelius et al. 2024; Strange 2024; LaGrandeur 2024). Researchers continue to point to recurring problems

DOI: 10.4324/9781042010912-1

such as dependence on massive datasets, limited capacity to operate reliably beyond narrowly trained contexts, opacity, disembodiment, and hallucinations (Xu et al. 2024; Maggiori 2023; Colbrook et al. 2022).

At the same time, the broader development and deployment of contemporary AI depend on extensive societal and material infrastructures that generate a range of social, cultural and ecological concerns, including exploitative labor practices, escalating environmental costs tied to large-scale model training (Crawford 2021; Budennyy et al. 2022), synthetic information pollution and declining content quality online (Martínez et al. 2023), expanding surveillance architectures (Zuboff 2019), growing social inequality (Eubanks 2018) and forms of cultural homogenization driven by large-scale generative systems (Bommasani et al. 2022).

Together, these technical limitations and broader societal consequences increasingly challenge the idea that contemporary AI systems are simply progressing toward seamless technological mastery. Yet for the present study, the central issue is not that AI encounters persistent limitations, but that these limitations and concerns appear to do remarkably little to diminish belief in AI's broader transformative potential. Even in what some describe as a "post-AI-hype" era (Munn 2023; LaGrandeur 2024), we are by no means living in a post-AI world. This raises the central question of this book: Why do such technological promises remain compelling despite the visible shortcomings and tensions surrounding contemporary AI systems? Rather than explaining this persistence primarily in technical or economic terms, this study examines how contemporary technological promises become bound up with questions of human orientation, uncertainty and self-understanding.

Addressing this question requires moving beyond AI understood as an isolated technology. Its promises, limitations and effects are inseparable from the data environments, algorithmic infrastructures and platform logics in which it is embedded and through which it operates. The apparent power of contemporary AI depends on architectures of data extraction, algorithmic sorting and real-time feedback mechanisms. Understanding AI therefore requires a broader analysis of the technological environments that sustain it.

Throughout this book, I use the term "technological environments" to refer to the constellation of data-driven, algorithmic, and AI-based systems that structure and mediate desire. The term "algorithmic environments" refers more specifically to those technological environments insofar as they operate through data processing, algorithmic sorting and feedback mechanisms that organize interaction and self-formation. AI does not stand outside this broader constellation; rather, it represents its most recent and perhaps most persuasive articulation, appearing uniquely capable of promising orientation, optimization and even salvation.

This dynamic is not entirely new. Earlier technological and scientific projects have carried similar promises of self-knowledge and mastery. The Human Genome Project promised to reveal the biological code of who we are, offering the prospect of complete genetic self-transparency and the elimination of disease (Rose 2007). Likewise, the decade of the brain suggested that mapping neural activity would grant unprecedented clarity about emotions, decisions and mental disorders, while the decade of the mind aimed to decode the mechanisms of thought, perception and identity (Abi-Rached and Rose 2010a, 2010b). Similar promises of mastery also shaped broader technological imaginaries surrounding nanotechnology, genetic enhancement and other visions of overcoming biological and cognitive limits through technological progress.

Contemporary technological environments shaped by algorithmic and AI-driven data inherit this trajectory, yet they differ in one crucial respect: they are interactive, adaptive and embedded in everyday life. Through continuous feedback loops, personalized recommendations and predictive interfaces, they do not merely promise transformation; they stage it in real time. They simulate a stable and knowable self whose desires appear consistent, predictable and already understood, transforming uncertainty into apparent clarity while masking what remains unresolved. In this sense, contemporary technological enviroments are sites in which desire is not only expressed but increasingly engineered.

One influential explanation for the growing influence of technological environments centers on power. From Foucault's analysis of disciplinary regimes to Zuboff's theory of surveillance capitalism, scholars have shown how data technologies function as instruments of behavioral control and social ordering (Foucault 1977; Zuboff 2019). Within capitalist systems, these infrastructures shape conduct, predict preferences and steer decisions, often without users' explicit awareness. The promise of personalization masks an asymmetrical dynamic in which users are profiled and categorized while the systems themselves remain opaque. Such analyses offer important insight into how technological environments organize behavior, attention and social relations through increasingly pervasive forms of monitoring, prediction and behavioral influence.

Yet this explanation remains incomplete. It is implausible that the widespread appeal of contemporary technological environments can be explained solely through coercion, manipulation or behavioral steering. Large social and symbolic systems rarely sustain themselves through external power alone. Even when people are aware of surveillance, profiling or algorithmic influence, they often remain deeply invested in the very systems they critically reflect upon. Public debates, critical media coverage and academic analyses have made many of the risks visible, yet awareness rarely translates into disengagement. This suggests that the attraction of technological environments can be understood not only in terms of external mechanisms of control but also in relation to the forms of orientation, meaning and promise that subjects themselves seek within these systems.

This study approaches that attraction through the lens of Lacanian psychoanalysis. Rather than reducing technological attachment primarily to power or ideology, Lacan's account of the subject as constitutively split and driven by desire offers a way to understand why promises of coherence, optimization and meaning exert such a powerful appeal. Desire, in this view, is not a lack that can simply be filled by the right object or technology but a structural condition that continually seeks symbolic support. Read through this lens, technological environments do not merely impose fantasies from the outside; they also provide new surfaces onto which long-standing desires for recognition, stability and wholeness can be projected. What is increasingly at stake, I argue, is not only the capacity of technological systems to influence behavior but their growing role in organizing desire itself: an ongoing engineering of desire.

From this perspective, the appeal of AI lies not primarily in what it objectively delivers but in how technological environments resonate with enduring desires for certainty, orientation and meaning. Their significance lies in how they organize and sustain fantasies of coherence, stability and completion. The persistent attraction to AI reflects, I propose, the fantasy of wholeness: a future in which uncertainty, division and lack might finally be overcome through technological mastery.

Focusing on how data-driven systems resonate with structures of desire also brings another aspect into view. These technologies do not only obscure or distort; they can also stage and amplify the dynamics through which subjects seek recognition, orientation and consistency, particularly when their modes of operation become visible and open to reflection. In such moments, technological environments may expose how desire is addressed, shaped and sustained within them, rather than merely directing it from behind the scenes.

This dual character is crucial. On the one hand, technological environments risk reinforcing illusions of coherence that invite subjects to deny their own fundamental indeterminacy and dependence, encouraging forms of self-relation shaped by algorithmic prediction and external validation. On the other hand, precisely because these environments can render their own mechanisms partially visible, they may open a space in which subjects recognize their division and uncertainty rather than conceal it. Such insight can open a more reflective relation to both traditional authorities and emerging digital "big Others," including the claims data-driven systems make about who we are and what we want. In this sense, technological environments are not merely dangerous or manipulative; they are also potentially illuminating. Lacanian psychoanalysis provides a framework for articulating this ambivalence by treating desire not as a problem to be solved but as a structural condition through which subjects relate to symbolic and technological environments.

To further demonstrate the relevance of this framework, I turn to Tinder as a paradigm case, not merely as a dating platform but as a medium of self-formation within contemporary technological environments. Because data-, algorithmic- and AI-driven systems function as enabling infrastructures embedded across many domains, Tinder is examined here not as an isolated object of study but as a revealing lens through which the dynamics of desire become especially visible. Once associated primarily with social awkwardness or loneliness, dating apps have become mainstream and increasingly shape the romantic lives of millions (Iqbal 2025; Wise 2023). Unlike many other forms of online activity, the search for a partner confronts subjects with a heightened degree of existential uncertainty: questions of identity, recognition, intimacy and lack move to the foreground, while the hope persists that the right encounter might resolve not only relational tensions but also deeper struggles within the self. Dating apps intensify this paradox. Through curated profiles, algorithmic suggestions and continuous feedback loops, desire is organized and reflected back to the user in ways that appear to offer self-knowledge and direction. The empirical observations discussed throughout the book remain illustrative rather than diagnostic, functioning as conceptual mirrors that clarify how subjects relate to technological promises of wholeness. It is precisely in this context that divided subjectivity becomes most visible and most vulnerable, as technological environments promise coherence and recognition while simultaneously shaping how users come to understand who they are and what they want.

The goal of this study is both descriptive and normative. Descriptively, it examines how technological environments structure desire and co-shape subjectivity, illustrated through the paradigm case of Tinder. Normatively, it asks whether these technologies enable a reflective engagement with lack and uncertainty or instead strengthen and sustain illusions of certainty and wholeness. Following Lacan's view of the subject as inherently split, the central question becomes: What forms of subjectivity do data-, algorithm- and AI-driven technologies produce through the structuring of desire, and do they support or obstruct our capacity to confront the constitutive lack at the heart of the human condition?

The book is structured into seven chapters. Chapter 2 develops the concept of algorithmic environments and shows how data-driven technologies organize social and intimate life and structure desire, shifting the analysis toward subjectivity within philosophy of technology. Chapter 3 introduces a Lacanian account of desire and subjectivity as the book's conceptual framework. Chapter 4 examines how algorithmic environments displace symbolic structures and reshape subject formation. Chapter 5 analyzes how technological environments stage promises of coherence and wholeness, and how subjects, structured along different clinical configurations, take up positions in relation to these promises, with Tinder as a paradigm case. Chapter 6 turns to design, exploring how technological environments might foster singularity rather than obscure structural lack. Chapter 7 concludes by reflecting on the broader existential promise and ambivalence of contemporary technological environments.

2 Technological Environments and the Formation of Desire

This chapter examines how technological environments shape the conditions under which desire is formed. It shows how data-driven and algorithmic systems not only influence behavior but increasingly structure how desire arises, takes form and is sustained.

The argument unfolds in three steps. First, it analyzes how technological environments permeate everyday life. Second, it explores a shift from theories of motivation to a focus on desire. Third, it shows how these environments move beyond behavioral steering toward the structuring of subjectivity, preparing the ground for the Lacanian framework developed in the next chapter.

Living in Technological Environments

The Intimate Reach of Technological Environments

Technology has become a pervasive force shaping nearly every aspect of contemporary life. It structures material, economic and social environments, from infrastructure and supply chain networks to financial transactions and workplace interactions, while extending deeply into personal and intimate domains such as friendship, romance and self-expression. The symbolic reinterpretation of Maslow's hierarchy of needs, humorously depicted in drawings where Wi-Fi appears even lower – and thus more basic – than food and water, does not simply exaggerate technological dependence. It points to a more fundamental shift: technology no longer merely supports the satisfaction of needs but increasingly constitutes the environment within which needs, wishes and desires arise, take form and are experienced.

Although ideology, politics and religion have long shaped both inner and outer life, technology has become a particularly dominant force, especially with the rise of information technologies in domestic spaces. Devices such as desktops, laptops, tablets and smartphones have become integral

DOI: 10.4324/9781042010912-2

to daily life. Smartphones, in particular, function as extensions of the body and mind, mediating access to information and structuring engagement with the world. Digital platforms now regulate an increasing share of economic, social and personal interactions, providing the infrastructure for activities such as banking, consumption, maintaining relationships and seeking romantic partners.

Within this broad landscape, the present study focuses specifically on data-driven and algorithmic technologies. To clarify this scope, several layers must be distinguished. Digital platforms function as sociotechnical interfaces through which interactions are organized. Data-driven systems collect and process large-scale datasets. Algorithmic technologies operate within these systems as procedures that sort, recommend and structure patterns of visibility and action. Artificial intelligence refers to configurations of these technologies that learn from data and adapt dynamically. Together, these layers form technological environments: structured constellations rather than isolated tools.

These environments operate through continuous data extraction and analysis. In order to provide services and maximize profits, platforms collect vast amounts of data to map behavior, anticipate actions and influence choices, often without users' explicit awareness. Users are gradually nudged to transfer activities previously conducted offline into these environments. As a result, algorithmic technologies influence not only how individuals act but also how they perceive themselves and shape their inner lives. They do not merely support desires; they increasingly structure and generate them.

This transformation becomes particularly visible when technological environments are understood not as discrete tools but as continuous infrastructures of interaction. Embedded in sensor-rich ecosystems, interconnected across networks and linked to remote digital infrastructures, these systems enable ongoing data collection and real-time responsiveness. Interaction is no longer episodic but continuous, extending across contexts, institutions and moments of everyday life. As a result, technological environments are not simply used; they are lived in (Aydin et al. 2019).

Predicting, Nudging and Behavioral Steering

The continuous and interconnected character of technological environments enables a shift from passive observation to active intervention. Because interactions are constantly registered and processed, these environments do not merely respond to behavior but increasingly anticipate and shape it. Prediction and influence thus become structurally intertwined: the more behavior can be tracked in real time, the more it can be steered as it unfolds.

Data mining refers to the process through which organizations detect and analyze patterns in data to derive insights aligned with commercial or public objectives. Advances in artificial intelligence have significantly expanded this capacity. Machine learning and deep learning techniques enable the transformation of raw data into predictions and adaptive responses through processes such as classification, clustering, regression, and long-term memory processing. These processes underpin algorithmic and AI-driven technologies.

Despite these developments, important limitations remain. Even under conditions of extensive data availability, AI systems struggle with generalization, the ability to apply learned knowledge to unfamiliar situations. Marcus (2018, 17) emphasizes that deep learning systems often fail outside their training data. While hybrid models may improve performance, these limitations indicate that algorithmic technologies do not simply predict behavior through neutral observation.

These limitations point toward an alternative explanation: predictive success increasingly depends on continuous monitoring and behavioral steering. Large-scale data collection enables technological environments to intervene directly in patterns of action. As Shoshana Zuboff (2019, 203) argues, ubiquitous computing functions not only as a knowing machine but also as an actuating one, shaping behavior to produce greater certainty.

A particularly clear illustration of this shift is the emergence of digital twins. Through the integration of multiple data sources and AI-driven modeling, systems generate continuously updated digital counterparts of objects, infrastructures and individuals, enabling ongoing monitoring, prediction and adjustment. Technological environments therefore no longer merely represent reality but actively participate in shaping it.

These developments have generated debate about nudging. Thaler and Sunstein (2008, 2021) argue that nudging can be ethically defensible as libertarian paternalism, while critics emphasize asymmetries of power. Zuboff (2019) argues that data-driven behavioral steering undermines autonomy (Kavenna 2019; Jackson 2021).

The question arises whether this represents a radical transformation or an intensification of existing practices. Historically, institutions have always guided behavior (Lovallo and Webb 2011). Acknowledging these continuities does not imply determinism. Individuals retain the capacity for critical reflection and self-critical distance. Aydin (2021) shows how long-term ideals can enable subjects to resist technological pressures and sustain agency within technological environments. Yet framing the issue in terms of continuity versus novelty remains insufficient. The more fundamental question is why subjects remain receptive to such influence at all.

Why Subjects Remain Receptive

The primary aim of this research is not to take a position for or against data mining, nudging or digital twins based on concerns about power asymmetries, privacy or freedom. Instead, the focus lies on understanding why and how subjects remain susceptible to technological influence in the first place. This requires insight into how subjects are always already shaped by their environments, which today increasingly take the form of data-driven and algorithmically structured technological environments. What is needed, therefore, is a theory of subjectivity capable of accounting for a world saturated with technological mediation.

Questions about how environments and technologies shape human beings have been explored from multiple theoretical perspectives. Many existing studies focus primarily on observable behavioral effects. Economists, sociologists, psychologists and other social scientists investigate how technological tools guide behavior through quantitative and qualitative research. Large-scale data collection, first through analog systems and later through digital infrastructures, has significantly expanded the capacity to identify patterns linking technological environments to behavioral change.

A second line of research examines the technical characteristics of algorithmic technologies themselves. A central concern here is the increasing opacity of AI systems. As technological environments grow more complex, it becomes increasingly difficult to understand how behavioral profiles and informational representations are constructed. In supervised machine learning, human guidance remains partially present. In unsupervised learning, however, pattern detection increasingly occurs without predefined human criteria. With deep learning, the training process itself becomes opaque, as multilayered computational structures generate outcomes that exceed human interpretability and reproducibility.

Proposed responses to this "black box" problem typically emphasize technical solutions: improving explainability, keeping humans in or on the loop or enhancing transparency and privacy protections through optimization and data filtering. While such approaches contribute valuable insights into algorithmic design and governance, they remain limited to external descriptions of technological mechanisms and their behavioral consequences. They do not explain why subjects remain receptive to technological influence even when these mechanisms are widely known and openly discussed.

This limitation points toward another black box, not technological but subjective. How is it possible that individuals continue to engage with technological environments despite awareness of their commercial logic and behavioral steering? What dynamics within subjectivity mediate the appeal of technological environments, sustain receptivity to algorithmic guidance and enable behavioral adaptation?

Addressing these questions requires moving beyond technical accounts and statistical correlations. Insight is needed into the affective and existential dimensions through which technological environments enter into conduct and shape experience from within. Only by examining this other black box, the structure of subjectivity itself, can we begin to understand how technological environments exert their influence and why that influence persists.

From Motivation to Desire

Competing Accounts of What Drives Behavior

The preceding section showed that accounts of technological influence tend to focus on behavior: how actions are predicted, nudged or steered. What remains insufficiently addressed is not how behavior is guided but what makes such guidance effective in the first place. Why are subjects responsive to these interventions at all? To answer this question, a shift is required from behavior to what drives it. Dominant accounts of motivation provide important insights, but they remain limited for this purpose: they explain how behavior can be directed, not why subjects remain invested in that direction.

What drives human behavior? A wide range of theories have been developed to answer this question (Ryan et al. 2019; Bandhu et al. 2024). These include hedonic motivation theories (traced back to the ancient Greeks), instinct theory (Wundt, late 1800s), behaviorisms (Pavlov, Watson, Skinner, Thorndike, late 1800s), goal-directed behavior theories (Craig, 1910s), Maslow's hierarchy of needs (Maslow, 1940s), social influence theories (Deutsch, 1950s), needs theories addressing achievement, affiliation, power and recognition (McClelland, Marlowe, 1960s), reward theories (various, 1970s), hedonic psychology (Kahneman, 1990s), the 6 Basic Desires theory (Reiss, 1990s), and situated motivation (Paris, 1990s).

Despite their diversity, these approaches converge on a shared intuition: behavior is propelled by identifiable forces, understood as either needs, drives, incentives or goals. Roughly, these theories can be grouped into four perspectives. Some emphasize external objects or goals toward which behavior is directed. Others stress situational factors that enable or constrain action. A third group locates the driver within the subject, in primary or secondary needs (Murray 1938). Interactionist approaches combine these dimensions, treating behavior as the outcome of their interplay.

These frameworks illuminate important aspects of human conduct. They show how behavior can be explained, predicted and, to a certain extent, influenced. At the same time, their explanatory power remains tied to observable patterns of action and identifiable motivational states.

What they do not yet account for is a more elusive dimension: how subjects become oriented toward certain objects in the first place, why they remain invested in these orientations, and why satisfaction repeatedly fails to resolve this investment.

In this sense, these theories clarify what moves behavior, but they are less equipped to explain what disposes subjects to engage. This limitation is not a flaw in the theories themselves; it reflects the level at which they operate. They remain within a framework in which what drives behavior is, in principle, identifiable and satisfiable. Precisely this assumption becomes problematic when explaining why subjects remain engaged in technological environments that promise fulfillment yet repeatedly defer it. To understand this persistence, a further conceptual step is required.

Theories of Desire

Because desire plays a central role in this study, it is useful to briefly examine influential theories of desire. The aim is not to reject these accounts but to clarify what they capture and where their explanatory scope proves insufficient for the present analysis.

Many influential theories define desire through its observable effects. Action-based theories (Anscombe 2000; Smith 1987, 1994), for instance, understand desire primarily as a disposition to act. Feeling or thinking are treated as secondary. This approach captures the close link between desire and action, but it risks conflating desire with other motivational states, since a desire does not always result in action, and action can arise from multiple sources (Davis 1984; Marks 1986).

Pleasure-based theories define desire through enjoyment or anticipated satisfaction (Schueler 1995; Vadas 1984). These accounts illuminate the affective dimension of desire, yet they struggle to explain why desires often persist even when they are not pleasurable, or why pleasure may follow rather than constitute desire (Davis 1984; Schroeder 2004).

Good-based theories link desire to value judgments, suggesting that to desire p is to judge p as good (Stampe 1987; Oddie 2005). Variants refine this by framing desire as the perception of goodness. These accounts clarify the normative dimension of desire but face difficulties in cases where individuals desire what they explicitly judge to be harmful, or in explaining desire in nonhuman animals. Related judgment-based approaches emphasize attention (Scanlon 1998), yet attention may be directed toward objects or experiences that are not structured as reasons (McDaniel and Bradley 2008), thereby weakening the link between desire and rational evaluation.

Biological and neuroscientific accounts locate desire in bodily and neural processes, such as dopamine signaling or opioid activity (Malenka et al. 2009, 147–148; Berridge and Kringelbach 2015). These models provide important insights into mechanisms of motivation and reward, but they tend to bracket the experiential and relational dimensions through which desire is lived (Brook 2006; Latham 2006).

Holistic theories attempt to combine multiple features (Lewis 1972; Davidson 1980), while further distinctions address intrinsic and instrumental desires (Frankfurt 1971, 1999; Arpaly and Schroeder 2014, 6), their strength (Von Neumann and Morgenstern 1944) or their temporal status (Hulse, Read and Schroeder 2004). These refinements enrich the conceptual landscape but struggle to specify which features are essential or how many are required, thereby leaving unresolved the broader question of what unifies these accounts of desire.

Across these approaches, desire is consistently explained through something else: action, pleasure, judgment, biological function, or evaluative states. Each theory captures a dimension of desire, and together they form a rich and nuanced field. At the same time, they share an underlying assumption: that desire can in principle be grounded in identifiable features or processes. For the purposes of the present analysis, this shared assumption leaves a crucial question open. It does not explain why desire persists beyond satisfaction, why it attaches itself to ever new objects, or why subjects remain invested even when promised fulfillment repeatedly fails to materialize.

Desire must therefore be approached not through its effects or correlates alone but at the level of its structure.

Desire as Structural Lack

This study adopts such a shift by approaching desire as a structural condition rather than a derivative phenomenon. As Lacan writes, "Desire, a function central to all human experience, is the desire for nothing nameable … and lies at the origin of every variety of animation" (Lacan 1991, Sem II, 223–224).

Desire, in this sense, cannot be reduced to action, pleasure, judgment or biological function. It is not one element among others, but the condition that renders these possible. It is not a thing but a no-thing: a structural lack. Crucially, this lack is not the absence of a particular object but a lack inherent to being itself: "This lack is the lack of being properly speaking … It is only ever represented as a reflection on a veil" (Lacan 1991, Sem II, 223).

From this perspective, desire is not oriented toward fulfillment in the straightforward sense assumed by many motivational theories. It is sustained by a fundamental noncoincidence with itself. As Lacan puts it, "Desire is a relation of being to lack" (Lacan 1991, Sem II, 223). What drives behavior is therefore not the pursuit of satisfiable ends but a structural condition that no satisfaction can resolve.

This does not contradict the insights of earlier theories; it reframes their scope. Needs can be satisfied, rewards obtained, goals achieved. Yet none of these exhaust desire. Even when what is sought is attained, something remains unsettled. Desire persists not because it has not yet found the right object but because it cannot be resolved by any object. It is sustained by this impossibility. This persistence becomes crucial for understanding how subjects remain invested in technological environments that repeatedly promise completion without delivering it.

The shift from motivation to desire thus introduces a different level of analysis. If desire is structural rather than reducible to identifiable drivers, then the question of technological influence must also be reformulated. It is no longer sufficient to ask how technologies steer behavior. The more basic question is how they engage with and operate within the structure of desire itself.

Desire, Subjectivity and Algorithmic Environments

Subjectivity as Structural Lack

Subjectivity must be understood in light of this structure of desire. If desire is a relation of being to lack, then subjectivity is not a stable substance but emerges through this lack. As Lacan puts it, "Being comes into existence as an exact function of this lack. Being attains a sense of self in relation to being as a function of this lack, in the experience of desire" (Lacan 1991, Sem II, 223–224). In this sense, the subject is not something that has desire; it is constituted through it. Lacan therefore appears to revise the Cartesian cogito: "'Desidero is the Freudian Cogito'" (Lacan 1977, Sem XI, 154).

This view does not present an overly cheerful outlook on life. It clarifies why satisfaction does not resolve the tensions of subjectivity, a point captured in various forms in the works of Oscar Wilde and George Bernard Shaw: "There are only two tragedies. One is not getting what one wants, and the other is getting it" (Wilde 1892); "There are two tragedies in life. One is to lose your heart's desire. The other is to gain it" (Shaw 1903). These formulations capture the paradox that satisfaction does not resolve the tension at the heart of subjectivity, leaving something structurally unsettled.

At the same time, this perspective should not be mistaken for a universal empirical claim. Life is not always tragic, and its difficulty varies across individuals and situations. Extensive empirical research on desire and happiness complicates any straightforwardly tragic reading. The point is not that all experience is marked by suffering but that the subject is structured by a fundamental noncoincidence with itself.

For Lacan, this entails an ontology without substance. As Jacques-Alain Miller observes, Lacan "inscribed his ontology within Freud's attempt to give body to psychical reality without substantifying it" (Miller May 11, 2011). The subject is not a fixed entity but a process, a becoming structured by an irreducible insufficiency. To be a subject is not to coincide with oneself but to persist in a relation to what one lacks.

Because desire cannot be made into a substance, it cannot be fully represented or brought to consciousness without distortion. It belongs to the order of the unconscious. Attempts to define the metaphysical essence of the subject by specifying what it is or wants to be therefore miss their object. The subject does not have desire; the subject is desire.

In this respect, Lacan aligns himself with a long tradition of philosophical thought that challenges the notion of the subject as a fixed substance. Most prominently, his view resonates with Hegel's claim that "substance is being which is in truth subject" (Hegel 2018, 12). Traces of Nietzsche are also visible, where the human being is understood not as a being but as a becoming, the "not yet determined animal" (Nietzsche 2002, 36; Aydin 2007). Perhaps even more explicitly, Lacan's view echoes Sartre's conception of human existence as grounded in nothingness: "[n]othingness lies coiled in the heart of being" (Sartre 2003, 45). Although these affinities are clear, Lacan articulates this condition within a psychoanalytic framework, emphasizing the structural role of desire and lack.

Crucially, this subjective condition is not formed in isolation. Desire is always mdiated through relations to others and to symbolic structures. As Lacan famously puts it, "Man's desire is the desire of the Other" (Lacan 1977, Sem XI, 235). Contemporary technological environments therefore play an increasingly decisive role in shaping how subjects relate to this lack. Data-driven and algorithmic technologies cannot be reduced to influencing behavior externally; they participate in structuring how subjects interpret dissatisfaction, recognition, and relational possibilities. This raises the question of how such structurally desiring subjects are shaped within contemporary technological environments.

From Behavioral Steering to the Structuring of Desire

If subjectivity is structured by desire, the question arises how this structure becomes a site of intervention. Marketing, advertising, and digital platforms increasingly draw on psychological insights to shape and sustain desire in order to achieve specific outcomes. Conceptions of desire similar to those found in Lacan resonate in fields concerned with behavioral influence. Lavidge and Steiner (1961), for instance, argue in their Hierarchy of Effects Theory that after capturing attention and interest, consumer desire must be continually fueled, illustrating how technological environments actively cultivate a sense of lack or wanting.

Earlier discussions of nudging and data mining showed how technological environments steer behavior through interface design, choice architecture, and continuous feedback. What is at stake, however, is not simply that these environments influence actions but that they operate within and through the structure of desire itself. They cannot be reduced to influencing behavior. Where earlier analyses emphasized behavioral control, the present discussion shifts to the structure through which behavior becomes meaningful and directed. Digital environments do not merely present options; they organize the field in which subjects search for recognition, orientation and coherence.

Because digital interfaces can be continuously monitored and adjusted through data mining, behavioral influence becomes more adaptive and responsive than in physical environments. Practices of digital nudging (Weinmann et al. 2016a, 2016b) therefore mark not only a technological development but a transformation in how desire is engaged and modulated. The distinction is crucial: influencing behavior operates at the level of choice, whereas structuring desire operates at the level of subject formation.

Thaler and Sunstein's notion of libertarian paternalism (2008, p. 5; see also 2003) frames nudging as a legitimate attempt to guide individuals toward choices that improve their well-being. Such approaches are illuminating but remain largely behaviorist or rationalist. They explain how people can be guided but not why subjects remain receptive to guidance even when its mechanisms are widely known. This limitation reflects their level of analysis: they address behavior without fully accounting for the structure of desire that sustains engagement. This gap points back to the ways in which technological environments resonate with the subject's search for completion and certainty.

This dynamic becomes most visible in domains where desire is particularly exposed. One such privileged site is the search for a partner. Here, questions of recognition, identity and lack come to the foreground. Tinder can therefore be approached not simply as a platform among others but as a condensed technological environment in which the structuring of desire becomes especially visible.

Within Tinder, algorithmic sorting, interface design and continuous feedback loops converge around the organization of desire. Profiles, matches and recommendations do not merely influence isolated choices; they shape anticipation, comparison and expectation. What appears as a sequence of individual decisions is inseparable from a technological arrangement that continuously modulates how desire is directed and sustained.

Seen in this way, Tinder does not simply exemplify an intensified form of behavioral steering; it reveals how technological environments operate at the level of desire itself. They structure how subjects relate to their lack, how they seek recognition, and how they interpret what they want. The question therefore is not only how platforms influence behavior but how they engage with the conditions under which desire takes shape.

To analyze this transformation, a theory of desire as structural lack is required. The next chapter develops such an account through Lacanian psychoanalysis, showing how desire is constituted through lack, mediated by the Other and sustained through structures that no object can resolve.

3 A Lacanian Account of Desire

This chapter develops a Lacanian account of desire, showing how the subject is constituted through lack rather than guided by stable needs or goals. Desire is not a property of the subject but the structural condition that animates and divides it, shaping its relation to itself, to others and to the symbolic order. By foregrounding the interplay between lack and identification, the chapter explains why promises of coherence, recognition and fulfillment remain compelling for a subject that does not coincide with itself. It also provides the conceptual coordinates for analyzing how technological environments reshape the relation between subjectivity, lack and the promise of fulfillment.

The chapter proceeds in three steps. First, it shows how subjectivity emerges through need, demand and desire, structured by the Real, the Imaginary and the Symbolic. Second, it develops the object of desire through the notion of *object a* and its relation to others and the Other. Third, it examines the divided subject of desire, its clinical structures and how each confronts the question of what it wants.

Becoming a Subject Through Need, Demand and Desire

The Imaginary, the Symbolic and the Real

Lacan distinguishes desire from related notions such as need and demand, situating them within three registers of existence: the Imaginary, the Symbolic and the Real. The register of the *Imaginary* is associated with the subject's earliest forms of identification, primarily through the experience of the mirror stage. When a child recognizes themselves in a mirror, or, more abstractly, in another person, a coherent self image or identity begins to form. However, this identity is illusory, as it is based on an external image rather than a complete inner sense of self. On the one hand, the self feels fragmented and incoherent; on the other, this fragmentation is masked by imaginary identifications. Others act as mirrors, offering affirmations such as "Look at you, what a beautiful person," or

DOI: 10.4324/9781042010912-3

"Yes, that's you, you're an amazing soccer player, maybe even better than Messi." Imaginary identification is accompanied by the pursuit of an ideal I, fully merged with the coherent and idealized images projected onto us by others. Despite these images coming from others, we cling to the idea that they are expressions of our own inner beliefs. We hold on to the illusion of being self-sufficient and autonomous, or at least capable of achieving autonomy. Paradoxically, even someone who wants to look like Jennifer Lopez can say: "One more operation and I'll look exactly like I really am."

The *Symbolic* represents the order of language, customs, rules, and cultural laws. Through symbolic structures, the subject is inscribed in a network of meanings, taking up a social identity through name, role and position. It is in the Symbolic register that the Name of the Father is established, a Lacanian term for the way prohibitions and institutional authority regulate the subject's desire and shape its identity. Aydin clarifies: "The Symbolic order, through language, is in essence a contract or tie between an individual and society" (Aydin 2021, 215). The imaginative constructs stemming from initial impulses are symbolized, regulated and organized by language and norms. While the Imaginary is bound by the need for recognition from others, in the Symbolic the subject must transcend its dyadic and narcissistic attachments, opening itself to relationships with society as a whole and submitting to social rules. Generally, Lacan refers to the symbolic function with the term "subject" (the subject of the unconscious), while le moi ("I" or "ego") designates the imaginary side (see Homer 2005).

The *Real* represents what escapes both the Symbolic and the Imaginary. It is compared with what cannot be processed within language, a grain of sand that makes the machine falter. Sometimes the Real is described as a state prior to individuation, before the self possesses an identity. However, since the subject comes into being through Symbolic structures, this "prior" should not be understood in a linear temporal sense. Recalcati explains: "The Real is an event that emerges from the Symbolic yet cannot be fully explained by the Symbolic itself" (Recalcati 2023, 52). The Real designates the limits of the Symbolic: it is the horizon of what resists symbolization. It signals both an absence and an excess, something irreducible that unsettles but also sustains the subject as a particular being. This residual dimension will become crucial later as a way to understand what resists organization and stabilization, especially within technological environments that promise orientation, coherence, and completion.

The three registers provide the basic coordinates for understanding how subjectivity emerges and is structured, as well as how desire takes shape within it. These registers are not linear-successive stages but enduring dimensions of subjectivity (see Lacan 1988 Sem II; Lacan 1997; Lacan 2006 Écrits; Elliott 2015; Laplanche and Pontalis 1973).

Need, Demand and Desire

Need, demand and desire articulate subject formation from a complementary perspective to that of the registers. Where the registers approach the subject from the side of its structuring conditions, these mechanisms express how the subject sustains and unfolds itself, each corresponding to one of the three registers.

Need is characterized as the primal urge of the newborn, who, after separation from the mother, experiences itself as lacking something beyond its immediate reach (Lacan 1991, Sem II, 223–224). The infant seeks satisfaction without conscious recognition of the separation between self and other. This rupture marks the beginning of individualization. Prior to this rupture, Lacan evokes a state of unity with the mother, sometimes compared to a "Garden of Eden," a state of fullness and completeness. Yet this wholeness is reconstructed only retroactively: even the idea that complete satisfaction once existed is itself a later symbolic construction. Fullness is defined negatively, through the absence of lack. This phase aligns with the Real, a limit category that can only be indicated through absence, loss or void.

The persistent urge to retrieve this lost wholeness structures human existence. Whether satisfying hunger, striving to run a marathon, or pursuing career success, subjects remain propelled by a fundamental drive to overcome the lack that defines them.

According to Lacan, *demand* emerges between 6 and 18 months, when the infant gradually develops a sense of self accompanied by an awareness of lost unity and nonseparation (Lacan 2006 Écrits, 75–81). The infant moves from insufficiency toward anticipation: still unable to be whole, it begins to anticipate wholeness, transitioning from the experience of a fragmented body toward what Lacan calls an orthopedic vision of its totality. This vision is "orthopedic" because the child relies on external supports to sustain coherence: crutches that enable standing, tools that compensate for deficiencies and, above all, parents who name and affirm the child's emerging identity (Lacan 2006 Écrits, 78).

In the Mirror stage (Lacan 2006 Écrits), Lacan shows how the child discovers and misrecognizes unity through "something else": its mirror image, the body of another or parental affirmation (see also Julien 1990, 43–51). The ego does not arise from an original inner core but through identification with external images. This development can only be reconstructed retrospectively; the ego is not given but produced relationally.

During this phase the child increasingly perceives itself as distinct from others while simultaneously demanding a return to lost unity. It attempts to overcome the vulnerability that accompanies individuation. Yet this return is impossible because the very condition for becoming a subject is the experience of lack. The transition from nature to culture requires the loss of unity with nature. By translating need into demand, however, an illusion emerges: that wholeness might still be retrieved. The ego thus develops within a fundamentally narcissistic structure, constructing fantasy images of itself and its ideal objects of desire. This phase corresponds to the Imaginary.

Demand, like the other mechanisms, is not merely a developmental stage but a structural dimension that persists throughout life (Moyaert 2011). To shield ourselves from the impossibility of completeness, we continuously misrecognize ourselves as autonomous and whole. Lack is reinterpreted as something that could in principle be overcome, and perfect images are projected as compensation (Lacan 2006 Écrits, 80). We identify with parental ambitions, imagine becoming pop stars or philosophers, or align ourselves with figures who promise fulfillment. Endless effort is invested in sustaining the illusion of eventual completion. Even burnout often generates a new fantasy: that rest and withdrawal will finally restore wholeness.

Self-identification through mirrors, supports and projections is inherently intersubjective and dyadic. Gradually, these processes enable the child to locate itself within a broader social and cultural order, forming a triadic configuration. Through language and other symbolic structures, the subject becomes capable of designating itself as "I" from a third-person perspective. The transition from demand to *desire* entails submission to sociolinguistic structures: customs, institutions, laws, norms and traditions. The ego becomes a subject through subjection to symbolic law; and because prohibition simultaneously implies the possibility of transgression, the "no" of society both constrains and fuels desire.

The impossibility of wholeness now appears within the Symbolic order. Desire is shaped not only by parental expectations but also by broader cultural frameworks whose ultimate meaning may assume metaphysical or religious form. In some traditions, fulfillment is projected into an afterlife, attached to a signifier that itself escapes full signification. This unfillable emptiness at the core of desire ensures that the subject continues to desire. Every fantasy and ideal construction ultimately fails because every object remains a substitute for something fundamentally beyond representation. The persistent misrecognition that fullness is attainable sustains the movement of desire.

The next section takes this structural gap as its point of departure and shows how it is precisely this gap that lends promises of coherence and completion their force. Desire persists as a remainder that cannot be resolved and, for that very reason, continually calls for fulfillment.

Desire as Remainder

Lacan sometimes enigmatically characterizes desire as the remainder left after subtracting need from demand. Where the previous section described how need, demand and desire emerge within the three registers, the present section clarifies their structural relation more analytically. In his words,

> Desire is neither the appetite for satisfaction nor the demand for love, but the difference that results from the subtraction of the first from the second, the very phenomenon of their splitting (Spaltung).
>
> (Lacan 2006 Écrits, 690–692)

Put simply, desire is what remains within a demand after a need has been fulfilled. Desire appears as a kind of residue, a remainder produced when a need is articulated, or "worded," into a demand. This articulation inevitably distorts the original need, omitting or displacing it, and thereby making complete fulfillment impossible.

Desire does not coincide with a specific need because even after a need is satisfied, there is always a remainder, something still unfulfilled. Desire is that "something" that prevents complete satisfaction. However, desire also does not coincide fully with demand. As Lacan points out, "Although it always shows through in demand, as we see here, desire is nevertheless beyond demand" (Lacan 2006 Écrits, 634). Whenever one articulates a desire through demand, one eventually discovers that what was truly desired differs from, or exceeds, what was asked for, thus keeping desire alive. In Lacan's words: "Demand by the necessities of its articulation deflects, changes, transposes need. There is therefore the possibility of a residue" (Lacan 2017 Sem V, 11).

Lacan offers several examples to illustrate how the articulation of need into demand necessarily produces an ambiguity that thwarts full satisfaction. He provocatively asks: If demand were simply about satisfying need, why, when clothing the naked, would it not be done with Christian Dior apparel? And why, when feeding the hungry, would it not involve letting them get drunk? (Lacan 2017 Sem V, 6). The point is that the object that fully satisfies demand is never unambiguously determined. What exactly is demanded when we ask for clothing, for food? When can we say that a need is fully met? How far must one go? There is a structural ambivalence in demand that cannot be eliminated.

Another example Lacan gives concerns the butcher's wife from Freud's *The Interpretation of Dreams*: "She loves caviar, but she doesn't want any. That's why she desires it" (Lacan 1977 Sem XI, 243). Here, Lacan shows that desire uses need as its vehicle. The butcher's wife craves caviar, articulates that craving in a demand, but does not act to satisfy it, thus preserving her desire (Lacan 2017 Sem V, 11–12). She seems to intuit that the worst thing one can do to desire is to attempt its full satisfaction.

However, Lacan's examples should not be misunderstood. It is not simply that people occasionally want more than they need, or that they consciously refuse fulfillment to preserve their desire. Rather, it is inherent to the structure of desire that it cannot be fulfilled. Desire's unfulfillability is not a choice but a structural necessity.

Lacan sometimes illustrates this by comparing desire to the linguistic mechanism of metonymy. Metonymy reflects the sliding of the signified beneath the signifier. In Lacan's words: "The function of desire is a last residuum of the effect of the signifier in the subject" (Lacan 1977 Sem XI, 154). Desire exists only in the movement from one signifier to another: because it slips from object to object, it has no particular object that can finally satisfy it. Thus, desire is always desire for something else. It is not that some people occasionally choose not to fulfill their wants; rather, any linguistic articulation of a need inevitably propels the subject beyond that particular need.

The relations between the Real, the Imaginary and the Symbolic, discussed in the previous section, shed further light on this. What is expressed in language (the Symbolic) can never fully correspond with the need at work "prior" to being articulated (the Real); what is articulated in a demand corresponds neither to the need on the subject's side nor to that which is acquired or offered to fulfill that need on the object's side. In entering language and the symbolic order, the subject is alienated from both biology and world. This creates a structural gap that can be viewed from two angles: on the one hand, there is a gap between the subject's need and the articulation of that need in a demand; on the other hand, there is a gap between the subject's demand and what is ultimately received as satisfaction.

Throughout his work, Lacan emphasizes that wherever we seek the object of desire, we encounter only lack, or at best a placeholder for lack. This placeholder refers back to an original, lost need: a need that, because of the passage from nature (the Real) to culture (the Imaginary and Symbolic), can no longer be fully articulated. Desire arises from this impossibility and is continuously fueled by it.

In the next section, I will elaborate further on this original object that fuels desire, what acan systematically discusses as *object a*, the object-cause of desire. I will also explore how the unfulfillability of desire, as clarified by the notion of *object a*, fundamentally shapes human subjectivity and conditions human existence.

The Object of Desire

Object a as the Object-Cause of Desire

The idea that desire is not fulfilled by any particular object, and thus is not ultimately directed toward something specific, is systematically developed by Lacan through his concept of *object a* (French: *objet petit a*). He distinguishes *object a* from an empirical object by characterizing it not as the object of desire but as the object-cause of desire. This distinction reflects the experience that we seem to strive on two levels: consciously seeking a particular object while unconsciously never being fully satisfied with it. *Object a* names both the force that awakens desire and the structural obstacle that prevents its complete fulfillment. It causes desire and simultaneously ensures that satisfaction remains out of reach.

An interpretation in Kantian terms may help clarify this dynamic. One could say that *object a* occupies a position at the intersection of the transcendental and the empirical. It allows everyday objects to shimmer with transcendental promise, elevating them beyond mere functionality, without ever delivering a final or complete fulfillment. In Kantian language, *object a* enables something of the noumenal to flash through the phenomenal without providing the stable unity of transcendental apperception. It loads objects with the hope of resolving existential and epistemic tensions, only to intensify desire by never fulfilling that hope.

Since the object-cause of desire can never fully coincide with a particular empirical object, Lacan emphasizes its negative character. It is not a positively identifiable thing but functions as a limit or obstacle to fulfillment. Žižek illustrates this with the example of Coke: "Coke has the paradoxical property that the more you drink the thirstier you get, the greater your need to drink more" (Žižek 2000, 19). Todd McGowan refines this distinction by separating the Coke itself as the object of desire from the Coke can as the object-cause of desire. The can, by limiting access, makes Coke desirable:

> When I have the object of desire [Coke] without the object-cause, without the limit [the can] that prevents me from fully having it, I cease to desire the object of desire, and it becomes a normal empirical object.
> (McGowan 2016, 64)

Thus, it is the barrier, the prohibition, that not only obstructs satisfaction but actively fuels and sustains desire. The "No" of the symbolic law, the No of the Father, becomes a necessary condition for the emergence of desire. Importantly, this limit is never confined to one material feature alone. In the case of Coke, not only the can but also factors such as unhealthy calories, caffeine, or the secrecy surrounding the formula function as obstacles that sustain fascination. The object that promises fulfillment is therefore always supported by an excess that keeps desire alive.

Contemporary consumer culture provides many comparable examples. High-caffeine, high-sugar or limited-edition drinks marketed through rumors of exclusivity or restriction illustrate how boundaries and prohibitions intensify attraction (think of Red Bull and Prime). The fascination does not stem from the empirical product itself but from the aura of inaccessibility that surrounds it. Yet these examples must not be taken too literally. The empirical object is never identical with *object a*. Earlier it was emphasized that *object a* refers to the elusive remainder that persists after a need, articulated in a demand, has been satisfied. What matters is not the material object itself but the function it comes to carry: that of prohibition, limitation, regulation and excitation.

This raises the question of where *object a* is situated within Lacan's three registers. In the Borromean knot of the Real, the Symbolic and the Imaginary, *object a* occupies a central position, tying the registers together. The Symbolic order comprises the network of language, law and social custom in which the subject is inscribed, while what Lacan calls the Big Other designates how this order is encountered: as an authoritative locus from which meaning and normativity appear to be articulated. Initiation into this order requires what Lacan calls symbolic castration: to become a social being, one must sacrifice "original jouissance" (Lacan 1992 Sem VII, 209). Jouissance here does not refer to ordinary pleasure but to an overwhelming excess that threatens both the subject and the social order. Lacan sometimes names this dimension Das Ding, the Thing that belongs to the Real and resists symbolization.

Lacan occasionally describes jouissance as a form of perfect satisfaction of the drive, yet he insists that actually attaining such satisfaction would be catastrophic for the organism and its environment. This is why he claims that every drive is, in a certain sense, a death drive. Žižek captures this relation succinctly: "Das Ding is the absolute void, the lethal abyss which swallows the subject; while objet petit a designates that which remains of the Thing after it has undergone the process of symbolization" (Žižek 1997, 105). Desire thus emerges not from access to fullness but from its structural deferral.

In this sense, Lacan often opposes jouissance to desire. Desire functions as a defense against the destabilizing pull of jouissance: "Desire is a defense, a defense against going beyond a limit in jouissance" (Lacan 2006 Écrits, 699). Through symbolic castration, jouissance is curtailed and defused, thereby evoking desire. As Lacan explains, "Castration means that jouissance has to be refused in order to be attained on the inverse scale of the Law of desire" (Lacan 2006 Écrits, 700). Crucially, the Symbolic does not simply follow the Real in a linear sequence. There was no fully enjoyed original jouissance prior to language; rather, the very restrictions of the Symbolic retroactively produce the fantasy of something lost. As Žižek puts it, *object a* "emerges as being-lost" (Žižek 1997, 15). It is the virtual trace of something that never existed as a complete presence.

Original jouissance is never possessed because the subject itself arises only through separation from an imagined unity with the (m)other. The subject emerges through mediation, through the impossibility of immediate satisfaction. From the beginning, pleasure is structured by lack. The subject desires substitute objects in the hope of regaining a fullness that was never fully present. Being a subject therefore means existing as a kind of nonbeing, a lack of being that continually seeks completion. It is not the absolute Other, *Das Ding*, that structures desire, but the partial remainder, *object a*, the little *a(utre)* that signals the symbolic order's inability to guarantee final meaning or satisfaction (Lacan 2014 Sem X, 124).

Object a belongs simultaneously to all three registers. It is Real insofar as it marks the lost remainder that sustains desire as long as it remains unconscious. It is Symbolic insofar as it arises through the operations of language that endlessly circle around what cannot be fully grasped. And it is Imaginary insofar as it appears as the missing piece the ego fantasizes it needs in order to become whole, a fantasy already rooted in the mirror stage. This triple status explains why Lacan's examples of *object a* often involve phenomena that hover between visibility and invisibility, inside and outside, presence and absence.

Perhaps the most illustrative example is the gaze, alongside other partial objects such as the voice, the breast or feces. The gaze cannot itself be seen, yet it exerts a powerful effect. It refers to the unsettling sensation of being looked at even when no observer is visible. As a manifestation of the Real Other, the gaze destabilizes orientation and confronts the subject with the question of how it appears to the Other. Even when one knows who is watching, one cannot see oneself as the Other sees. The gaze therefore provokes the question: "What do you want from me?" or "Where do I stand in relation to the Other's desire?" These are questions that resist definitive answers.

In this way, the gaze, as *object a*, sustains and fuels desire. It is not the object that one desires but the cause that makes desire circulate from one object to another in the hope that something might finally fill the structural lack that defines subjectivity and provide a final answer to what it really wants (see also Žižek 1997, 53).

Others as Objects of Desire

Object a functions as the cause of desire, rendering everyday objects mere substitutes for a lost object that never truly existed. A question that arises is how other people fit into this Lacanian framework. Does the desire for other people have a different structure than the desire for objects?

Following the line of thought so far, the basic structure remains the same. Like ordinary objects, other people can come to occupy the place of *object a*. This becomes particularly evident in the context of intimate relationships. The final chapter of Seminar XI, tellingly titled "In you more than you," opens with the striking formulation: "I love you, but, because inexplicably I love in you something more than you – the objet petit a – I mutilate you" (Lacan 1977 Sem XI, 263). From this perspective, interactions with others, including intimate and sexual relationships, are often structured by the search for *object a*, the elusive object-cause that appears to promise the resolution of the subject's lack. The other is not simply desired and loved for who he or she is but as a vehicle for something in the other that promises to resolve the subject's lack.

To sustain this promise, the partner is inevitably filtered through fantasy. Traits that support the fantasy of completeness are emphasized while others are ignored or bracketed. The romantic phrase "you make me complete" therefore acquires a less romantic meaning: the beloved becomes the screen onto which the subject projects the hope of overcoming its constitutive lack.

Yet because this lack is structural, no partner can ultimately occupy the place assigned to them in fantasy. The promise of completion that animates the relationship is therefore bound to fail. This is the background to Lacan's provocative claim that "there's no such thing as a sexual relationship" (Lacan 1998 Sem XX, 12). The claim does not deny the existence of intimate relations. Rather, it indicates that no relationship can fully realize the fantasy of perfect complementarity. Because *object a* is structurally unattainable, no partner can ultimately occupy the place of the lost object that desire seeks. The sublimity that partners acquire through their association with *object a* is therefore always provisional.

This becomes particularly visible when the fantasy that sustains desire begins to collapse. When traits that do not fit the sustaining fantasy become too visible to ignore, the partner loses the aura that once surrounded them and appears instead as an ordinary and imperfect person. In Lacan's words, "I give myself to you ... but this gift of my person ... is changed inexplicably into a gift of shit" (Lacan 1977 Sem XI, 268). Once the fantasy collapses, desire often shifts elsewhere, searching for another person who appears better suited to embody *object a*.

This logic is not confined to human relations; it also applies to everyday objects. The desire for Coke, to take up this example again, is sustained only under particular conditions. Coke retains its appeal when served cold and at the right moment; it quickly loses its allure when it becomes warm or flat. Similarly, if served early on a winter morning, it is unlikely to be experienced as desirable. Although it may seem awkward to compare a beverage with a partner, Lacan's framework deliberately invites such parallels. What matters is not the intrinsic nature of the object but the way it becomes invested with the promise of something more. As long as that promise is sustained, the object appears sublime. When the fantasy collapses, the same object appears banal or even repulsive.

Media stereotypes often reinforce and homogenize these fantasies of the perfect partner. Yet the key similarity between Coke and a partner lies in the fragile, reversible transition from the sublime to the mundane. A partner can suddenly lose their sublime status. Sometimes it is even the very traits that once seemed sublime that come to be perceived as vulgar, annoying, or inappropriate. When the fundamental fantasy can no longer be sustained, separation often seems inevitable. This also explains why, during and after a breakup, all the partner's traits that once were ignored are suddenly emphasized to rationalize the separation. And so the search for *object a* continues unabated.

Yet intimate relationships also differ from ordinary objects in an important respect. Phones, cars or beverages may temporarily function as stand-ins for *object a*, but they are not themselves structured by lack in the same way human beings are. A partner is not merely an object in the world but another subject whose own desire is equally structured by lack. Intimate relationships therefore involve a double encounter with desire: each partner approaches the other as a potential bearer of *object a* while simultaneously confronting the other's own lack and desire. This mutual opacity introduces a complexity absent from ordinary objects. A car does not desire us back, nor does it confront us with its own uncertainty about what it wants. In relationships between subjects, however, desire becomes entangled with the question of the other's desire. The subject is concerned not only with what it wants from the other but also with what the other wants from it and how it appears in the field of the other's desire.

Because another person is also a desiring subject, and thus appears capable of recognizing, responding to and completing us, intimate relationships carry a far greater existential weight than ordinary objects do. They promise not merely pleasure or utility but, more explicitly and convincingly, the possibility of overcoming lack. This expectation also introduces a specific risk: when the other is taken to resolve the subject's lack definitively, the structure of desire itself is misrecognized, and the relationship becomes burdened with an impossible demand.

For this reason, intimate relationships are a privileged site for the present analysis. Others appear capable not only of recognizing and responding to us but of completing us. Precisely this intensity makes this domain particularly revealing. If the structure of desire is misrecognized anywhere, it is here, where the expectation arises that another person might finally make one whole.

Desire as the Desire of the Other

If desire is structured by a lack that can never be fully resolved, it does not, on its own, indicate what is to be desired. The question therefore arises how desire nonetheless acquires direction. This direction emerges through its relation to others: desire does not unfold in isolation but is oriented through the field of the Other. As Lacan famously formulates it, "Man's desire is the desire of the Other" (Lacan 1977 Sem XI, 235). This formula complements the structural account developed so far: whereas the concept of *object a* explains why desire never reaches final satisfaction, the notion of the Other explains how it becomes directed and sustained within a social field. The subject does not simply pursue objects that seem capable of filling its lack but looks to others and to the symbolic order to determine which objects are worth desiring in the first place.

This dynamic can be understood in two closely related ways. First, we tend to desire what we suppose others desire. As Lacan puts it, the object of desire "is essentially an object desired by someone else," a process that renders objects comparable and exchangeable (Lacan in Furman and Levy 2003, 295–296). The value of what we desire does not reside in the object itself but is conferred upon it through the desire of others. This explains why radically different things become desirable in different contexts. It also helps explain why we wear what we wear, eat what we eat, take certain jobs and even choose one partner rather than another.

This first reading should not be reduced to simple imitation. It is not merely that we take over what others desire; rather, others function as a point of reference through which objects become desirable in the first place, conferring value and direction on what is to be desired.

At this point Lacan distinguishes between the other and the Other. The other refers to concrete individuals with whom we interact, while the Other designates the symbolic structures that organize social life: norms, institutions and cultural expectations. These dimensions are distinct but inseparable: the others we encounter are themselves shaped by the symbolic order, while the symbolic order becomes effective through these concrete relations. Initially, the self identifies with significant others, projecting onto itself, for example the ambitions of parents or the dreams and fantasies of peers. Gradually, however, the subject comes to orient itself toward what Lacan calls the Big Other, which represents the laws, ideals, and moral frameworks of a culture.

This account of why we desire what we desire is not detached from the discussion of *object a* but complements it. It helps explain why the search for the enigmatic lost object endures. Although we do not know how the objects we desire could ever bring us back to *object a*, fully satisfy us or make us whole, we often assume that others know. We see others passionately desiring certain things and imagine that they must know something we do not. This begins in early childhood, when children imitate their parents, and continues into adulthood, when the desires of neighbors, peers or public figures shape our own sense of what is worth pursuing.

Culture, with its rules, customs, doctrines and expectations, increasingly intrudes into life by indicating how it should be fulfilled. The social and cultural embeddedness of human beings thus brings with it a dependency that both instigates and structures desire. What the desire of the other or the Other actually yields remains enigmatic. Yet subjects often assume that the Other must know what is worth desiring. The more opaque and authoritative the Other appears, the more easily it functions as a presumed source of orientation. At the same time, because the desire of the Other can never be fully known, this supposed source of certainty also generates uncertainty. One may think here of the certainty some people claim to find in God and the despair the same figure evokes in others. From a Lacanian perspective, even God can function as an ultimate figure of the Other: a presumed locus that appears to know what should be desired while ultimately serving as another placeholder for *object a*.

The second reading of Lacan's maxim concerns desire as a demand for recognition. As Lacan puts it, to ask what the other desires is "the desire to have his desire recognised"; accordingly, "man's desire is alienated in the other's desire" (Lacan 2006 Écrits, 343). Desire is thus directed not only toward objects but also toward being recognized by the other or the Other. Understood in this way, a fundamental indeterminacy emerges: the subject cannot know what the Other wants from it, and therefore continues to address the Other with this question, keeping desire in motion. The subject is thus concerned not only with what it wants but with what it is for the Other, seeking recognition within a field whose expectations can never be fully known.

This dual structure produces a tension. On the one hand, the Other provides orientation and hope by presenting models of what counts as a meaningful life: laws, norms and ideals indicate which goals and forms of life are valued within a culture. On the other hand, these same structures impose demands and require conformity, shaping and constraining desire without ever resolving it. The subject is thus guided by the Other yet never definitively satisfied by it, remaining dependent on a source of orientation that cannot fully clarify what is to be desired.

Within this tension Lacan situates the problem of recognition. Desire is directed not only toward objects suggested by the Other but also toward being recognized by that Other. As he puts it, "the desire for recognition dominates the desire that is to be recognised, preserving it as such until it is recognised" (Lacan 2006 Écrits, 431). The decisive question therefore shifts: not what the object of desire is, but how the subject's desire is recognized within the field of the Other. Desiring what appears desirable to the Other and seeking recognition from the Other are thus two sides of the same movement, through which the subject's own desire is gradually formed rather than simply given.

Lacan is explicit about the Hegelian roots of this idea:

> Man's very desire is constituted, he tells us, under the sign of mediation: it is the desire to have one's desire recognised ... we find this anew in the whole development of his satisfaction, beginning with the conflict between master and slave, through the entire dialectic of labour.
> (Lacan 2006 Écrits, 182)

The process of discovering what the other desires, wants and demands is thus simultaneously a process of recognition through which the subject appropriates its own desire.

Applied to intimate relations, this dynamic becomes especially visible. If the other offers too little orientation, the subject becomes uncertain and no longer knows how to obtain the recognition it seeks. Yet if the other offers too much certainty, desire risks stagnating, and the subject risks being fully determined by the other's expectations. Nowhere is this tension more charged than in the search for a partner. Because intimate relations are invested with the hope that another person might give orientation to one's desire, the question of what the other wants acquires a distinctive existential weight.

Lacan illustrates this uncertainty through his well-known example of the praying mantis:

> I pictured myself faced with another animal, a real one this time, taken to be gigantic for the sake of the story, a praying mantis. Since I didn't know which mask I was wearing, you can easily imagine that I had some reason not to feel reassured in the event that, by chance, this mask might have been just what it took to lead my partner into some error as to my identity. The whole thing was well underscored by the fact that, as I confessed, I couldn't see my own image in the enigmatic mirror of the insect's ocular globe.
>
> (Lacan 2014 Sem X, 6)

Here Lacan magnifies the problem of not knowing what the Other wants. If I do not know which mask I am wearing, I do not know what I am for the Other, and therefore I do not know how the Other will relate to me or how I should relate to it. Because the subject discovers its own desire only through the desire of the Other, it can become uncertain about its own position within the field of the Other's desire. The question "What does the Other want from me?" thus becomes inseparable from the question of what I myself should want.

This uncertainty becomes particularly acute in intimate relations, where subjects seek recognition and orientation from another whose desire is itself opaque. Even when contemporary technological environments appear to organize this search by presenting potential partners through profiles, matches and algorithmic suggestions, the fundamental uncertainty remains. The subject must still interpret the desire of the other and determine how to position itself in relation to it.

The allegory of the praying mantis thus shows that the subject of desire cannot be understood independently of the relations through which it is mediated. The subject comes to know what it desires only by attempting to read the desire of the Other, yet that desire can never be fully known. Its position is therefore inseparable from the objects and others, as well as the networks, platforms and infrastructures, through which it takes shape. Desire is thus sustained between an object that cannot satisfy it and an Other that appears to give it direction. It is within this tension that the subject of desire emerges.

The Subject of Desire

Between Being and Nonbeing

The subject of desire cannot be understood apart from *object a* that causes it. Lacan stresses that "everything turns around the subject's relation to a" (Lacan 2014 Sem X, 112). Subject and *object a* are therefore not externally related but structurally intertwined: *object a* both sustains desire and marks the impossibility of its fulfillment. As the object-cause of desire, it reveals the subject as a lacking being, as well as a being that seeks to overcome its lack without ever succeeding. The subject seeks completion through objects, relationships and the other's desire, yet entry into the symbolic order entails the impossibility of direct and complete jouissance. What appears as a lost "part" is not something once possessed but a retroactively constructed loss that sustains desire. The promise of regaining it is therefore deceptive: to be a subject is to remain structured by a lack that cannot be overcome.

The strict correlation between the subject and *object a* as object-cause of desire is also emphasized by Žižek. In his account, this correlation makes otherness internal to subjectivity itself: the subject exists as a desiring being only insofar as it is not yet what it seeks to be, only insofar as it remains incomplete. Žižek articulates the paradox as follows:

> For Lacan, the subject ($ — the 'barred', empty subject) and the object-cause of its desire (the leftover which embodies the lack that 'is' the subject) are strictly correlative: there is a subject only in so far as there is some material stain leftover that resists subjectivization, a surplus in which, precisely, the subject cannot recognize itself. In other words, the paradox of the subject is that it exists only through its own radical impossibility, through a 'bone in the throat' that forever prevents it (the subject) from achieving its full ontological identity. So we have here the structure of the Moebius strip: the subject is correlative to the object, but in a negative way – subject and object can never 'meet'; they are in the same place, but on opposite sides of the Moebius strip.
>
> (Žižek 2000, 28)

This account clarifies what Lacan calls the barred or split subject. Crucially, this split does not consist of two positive aspects, such as what is made of the subject by others versus what the subject "really" is apart from them. That would presuppose the possibility of recovering an authentic core, which has no place in Lacan's view. Rather, the split consists in the division between being and nonbeing. Because *object a* is a residue of radical otherness, the subject exists only through its relation to a fundamental negation. It is not fully what it is, nor simply what it is not, but persists in the gap between the two. This lack propels it forward and prevents it from ever coinciding with itself.

This structure of existence through lack has far-reaching implications for how the subject relates to itself, to others and to the Other. Because the subject is constituted through a lack it cannot eliminate, it is continually driven to seek ways of overcoming or compensating for that lack. It invests in projects, relationships, identities and ambitions that promise to fill the gap that drives it forward. The subject pursues objects, builds networks and enters intimate relations in the hope of finding the missing part that would finally make it whole. In Lacan's terms, the subject exists only by virtue of this quest for *object a*: the elusive object that appears to promise the resolution of its lack while simultaneously sustaining the movement of desire that constitutes the subject itself.

Understanding the subject as existing through lack also clarifies Wilde's famous claim that there are two tragedies in life: not getting what one wants, and getting it. The subject is caught between these two poles. On the one hand, the subject cannot obtain the object that would finally resolve its lack. On the other hand, if such an object were truly obtained, if the missing part were definitively found, the very movement of desire that sustains the subject would come to an end. The subject exists only as a desiring being, as a being in pursuit of something it does not have and cannot be. An object, event, or partner that could truly close the gap and eliminate the subject's division would therefore threaten the very conditions of the subject's existence.

When such a situation appears to arise, it generates anxiety. One form this anxiety can take is what Lacan describes as a "lack of lack." Here the other seems to supplement the subject so completely that the distance required for desire disappears. The other anticipates and determines the subject's wishes even before the subject can articulate them. Instead of relating to the other as a separate being, the subject experiences a suffocating closeness in which it is absorbed by the other's presence. The space that normally sustains desire collapses, and with it the subject's ability to position itself in relation to the other.

In the Dutch film *De Beentjes van Sint Hildegard*, Herman Finkers illustrates how such a "lack of lack" can unfold in everyday life. In one scene, his wife asks him: "Do you have everything you want?" Finkers replies in dialect: "Gedda, you know that better than I do!" The remark is humorous, yet it reveals something unsettling. His wife appears to know him so completely that there is no room left for uncertainty or distance. She anticipates his wishes before he can articulate them himself. What looks like intimacy gradually becomes suffocating. If the other already knows what one wants, even before one can ask the question oneself, one's own desire – and with it one's subjectivity – begins to disappear. In response, Finkers starts behaving increasingly erratically, deliberately acting in unexpected ways simply to escape the role his wife has fixed for him. By making himself unpredictable he attempts to reintroduce a margin of otherness between them and to reclaim a space in which he can again appear as a subject. The scene suggests that some degree of distance or opacity between partners is not a failure of intimacy but a condition for sustaining both desire and subjectivity.

A second manifestation of this existential threat follows the opposite path: not from receiving too much but from receiving too little recognition. If the subject cannot obtain recognition from the other, the very coordinates through which it understands itself begin to collapse. Lacan's famous example of the praying mantis captures this situation vividly. In its attempt to become someone, the subject depends on recognition by the other. Yet when recognition fails, or when it becomes impossible to read what the other wants, the subject risks losing its orientation altogether. Not knowing what the other wants also means not knowing how to shape one's own position in relation to that desire.

Because the subject is structurally lacking, split and incomplete, it constantly turns to the other to discover what it should want and who it should be. It mirrors the other in order to locate its own desire. The man asks the woman what it means to be a man, and the woman asks the man what it means to be a woman. One might add that the nonbinary, by positioning itself in relation to the binary, poses the same question in a different way, and vice versa. In each case the subject seeks orientation in the other's desire. Yet because that desire can never be fully known, the question remains unresolved. Subjects repeatedly turn to others and the Other and ask, sometimes with increasing urgency, sometimes almost in despair: "Who am I?"

Clinical Structures as Responses to Lack

The previous section showed that the subject exists only as a desiring being, structurally split between being and nonbeing and propelled by the lack that *object a* embodies. This condition arises through entry into the symbolic order: in becoming inscribed in this order, the subject loses any direct, unmediated relation to the world and to itself and becomes dependent on others and on the Other for orientation and recognition. This mediation both constitutes and divides the subject, introducing a lack that cannot be overcome even as it is continually addressed in desire.

Others and the Other are therefore indispensable yet insufficient: they orient desire but cannot restore the immediacy they presuppose. The subject is thus situated between two limits: the absence of recognition, which threatens nonbeing; and the overwhelming presence of the Other, which threatens to absorb it completely.

Lacan's clinical structures articulate how the subject organizes its relation to the impossibility of an unmediated relation to itself, a lack that arises through its mediation by the Other. Psychosis, perversion and neurosis are not pathologies in a narrow sense but distinct structural responses to the loss introduced by symbolic mediation. Each structure positions the subject differently with respect to castration and lack: psychosis through foreclosure, perversion through disavowal and neurosis through repression.

Psychosis

One such configuration is *psychosis*. Here the symbolic mediation that normally introduces the subject into the order of language fails to take hold. A psychotic structure is characterized by the foreclosure of the Name-of-the-Father, which in Freudian terminology corresponds to what Freud called rejection (*Verwerfung*). Foreclosure is a specific form of negation in which the fundamental signifier that introduces the subject into the symbolic order is never integrated into the subject's symbolic universe. It is excluded from the symbolic order altogether.

To grasp the implications of this, Lacan's concept of the Name-of-the-Father must be clarified. It does not refer to an empirical father but to a fundamental signifier that anchors or "quilts" signifier and signified. It functions as a stabilizing point in language that organizes meaning, regulates the relation between desire and law and allows the subject to situate itself within a shared symbolic order. Through this signifier the subject can interpret what others want and position its own desire in relation to them.

In psychosis, this anchoring signifier is foreclosed. When the Name-of-the-Father would normally be called upon to stabilize meaning, nothing in the symbolic order answers that call. As Lacan puts it, "At the point at which the Name-of-the-Father is summoned … a pure and simple hole may thus answer in the Other" (Lacan 2006 Écrits, 465–466). Because this signifier is missing, the network that ordinarily links signifier and signified remains structurally incomplete. Experiences therefore lack the symbolic mediation that would situate them within a stable framework of meaning. Perceptions, thoughts and events still occur, but they cannot be securely interpreted or integrated.

What cannot be symbolically integrated may return from outside the symbolic order, often in the form of hallucinations or other intrusive phenomena (Laplanche and Pontalis 1973, 168). As a result, the subject lacks the coordinates that normally allow one to distinguish between imagination and reality and to situate its own desire in relation to that of others.

Vanheule (2011, 68) notes that the term "foreclosure" has legal origins. In legal contexts it refers to a situation in which a homeowner can no longer meet the obligations of a mortgage, allowing the lender to repossess the house. Lacan adopts this term metaphorically to describe a structural relation between the subject and the symbolic order. Whereas the paternal metaphor installs the subject within the symbolic order and allows it to inhabit its conventions, the psychotic remains excluded from this symbolic infrastructure. In this sense, the subject never becomes a "resident" within the symbolic house of language and law and cannot rely on it to organize experience or to situate itself among others.

This exclusion has direct implications for identity formation. Because the Name-of-the-Father normally regulates the desires of others and situates the subject within a shared symbolic network of meaning, its foreclosure leaves the subject without a stable framework for orientation. The interpretive process through which subjects read what others want and position their own desire in relation to it cannot properly take place. The desires of others do not appear as interpretable signals but remain opaque and unpredictable.

Vanheule (2011, 69) therefore observes that foreclosure undermines the experience of identity itself. Even doubt presupposes a minimal symbolic position from which it can arise. The psychotic lacks this anchoring and does not occupy a stable place within the symbolic network through which questions of identity normally emerge. As a result, questions such as "Who am I?" or "What do you want from me?" do not function as structuring questions within the psychotic register, because the symbolic framework within which they could be posed is itself missing.

The psychotic structure includes several forms, most notably paranoia and schizophrenia. In paranoia the subject often constructs elaborate interpretive frameworks in which meaning appears excessively stabilized. Because symbolic anchoring is foreclosed, the world may be experienced as saturated with hidden intentions or messages directed specifically at the subject. What appears as certainty is therefore not the resolution of doubt but an attempt to compensate for the absence of a stable symbolic framework (Lacan 2006 Écrits, 465–466; Lacan 1997 Sem III).

In schizophrenia the difficulty takes a different form. Rather than an excess of stabilization, signifiers tend to fragment and lose coherence. Language may become disorganized, associations unstable, and the subject may struggle to maintain a position from which experience can be interpreted. In both cases the subject's relation to desire and identity becomes precarious, as the symbolic coordinates that would ordinarily organize experience are missing.

Perversion

A second structural response to lack and castration takes the form of *perversion*. Unlike psychosis, it does not involve the rejection of the paternal law but is characterized by disavowal (*Verleugnung*). The pervert recognizes symbolic castration yet refuses its implication: that full jouissance and complete wholeness are impossible.

Rather than renouncing this impossibility, the pervert sustains the fantasy of full jouissance by interpreting the Law in a specific way. The Law is treated as an instruction: if followed precisely enough, satisfaction might still be achieved. As Clavreul (1980) notes, the tension between desire and Law is resolved by transforming desire into the rule that guides action. In this sense the pervert addresses the Other as if saying: your command is my wish.

This position reshapes the relation to the Other. The distinction between demand and desire collapses: what the Other demands is taken as a transparent expression of what it wants. The Other no longer appears as lacking or enigmatic but as determinate, and the subject positions itself as the object capable of fulfilling it. As Lacan puts it, "The subject here makes himself the instrument of the Other's jouissance" (Lacan 2006 Écrits, 320).

In occupying this position the subject secures its own satisfaction. By staging itself as the object that fulfills the Other's demand, it acquires a determinate place within the Other's desire and avoids the uncertainty that ordinarily sustains desire. Its satisfaction lies not beyond the Law but in enacting it as if it were fully coherent and satisfiable. In this way the pervert attempts to bypass the impossibility of jouissance by staging situations in which that impossibility appears suspended.

This organization removes the enigma that elsewhere characterizes the subject's relation to the Other. There is no open question of what the Other wants. The Other is reduced to a concrete other whose wishes can be satisfied, and desire is oriented toward a specific object that appears capable of filling that place.

The implications for subjectivity are decisive. The question "Who am I?" does not emerge as an open problem. Instead, the subject identifies with the object that completes the Other. This apparent clarity comes at a price: by fully occupying this role, the subject relinquishes the openness in which desire can emerge. Subjectivity is no longer organized around lack and questioning but around a fixed position within the Other's enjoyment. Rather than discovering what it wants through the enigmatic desire of the

Other, the subject assumes that this desire is already known and that its task is to embody the object that satisfies it.

The perverse structure appears in several recognizable forms, most notably fetishism, sadism and masochism. In fetishism the subject disavows symbolic castration by attaching a special status to a particular object. This object functions as a support that allows the subject to sustain the belief that nothing essential is missing, or that the lack introduced by castration can be bypassed. In this way the fetish stabilizes the subject's relation to desire without confronting its structural impossibility (Lacan 2006 Écrits, 319–324).

Sadism and masochism organize this logic differently while remaining structurally aligned. In sadism the subject positions itself as the agent of the Other's law, actively staging scenarios in which the Other's supposed demand for jouissance is imposed on the other. In masochism the subject instead positions itself as the object of the Other's law, offering itself as the site through which the Other's jouissance is realized. Where the sadist enacts, the masochist submits; yet in both cases the subject orchestrates the situation so that the Other's desire appears determinate and executable.

What appears as certainty about what is to be done thus functions as a defense against structural lack. Rather than confronting the impossibility introduced by castration, the subject sustains the illusion that this gap can be closed and that a form of wholeness might still be achieved (Lacan 2006 Écrits, 320; Lacan 1998 Sem XX).

Neurosis

A third response is *neurosis*. The neurotic structure is characterized by repression (*Verdrängung*). Repression does not exclude the Name-of-the-Father but integrates it into the symbolic order while pushing its implications out of consciousness. The impossibility introduced by symbolic castration is thus acknowledged yet not fully assumed, returning in the form of a persistent questioning of what the Other wants.

Neurosis is therefore structured by an unresolved relation to the Other. The subject encounters the Other as lacking and enigmatic, which means that its desire cannot be directly known or satisfied. As a result, the subject continually asks what the Other wants and how it should position itself in relation to that desire. Lacan accordingly describes neurosis as organized around a question addressed to the Other (Lacan 1997 Sem III, 174).

This distinguishes neurosis from the other structures. Unlike psychosis, the paternal metaphor is not foreclosed but operative, allowing the subject to inhabit a shared symbolic framework. And unlike perversion, the law is not treated as a transparent command that can simply be enacted. Instead, the ambiguity of the Other's desire is sustained. The subject neither loses the symbolic coordinates that organize experience nor resolves their uncertainty but remains caught within them.

From this follows neurosis's defining feature: doubt. The subject senses that the Other does not possess the answers it appears to promise, yet continues to seek them. In this respect, neurosis most closely reflects the general account of the subject developed earlier, namely as a divided being that depends on the Other for orientation while confronting a lack that cannot be resolved. The neurotic does not escape this tension but inhabits it in the form of ongoing questioning.

Since Lacan links the unconscious specifically to repression, and since repression is central to the constitution of the divided subject, neurosis comes closest to what may be called the ordinary condition of subjectivity in Lacanian terms. This claim requires qualification. It does not mean that psychosis and perversion lack subjectivity, but that subjectivity is configured there otherwise, through different relations to lack, castration and the Other.

This difference can be clarified in terms of alienation and separation. In neurosis, both are operative: the subject is constituted through its inscription in the symbolic order (alienation) and remains divided by its inability to coincide with the desire of the Other (separation). Neurosis thus most fully embodies the form of subjectivity developed throughout this chapter: a subject sustained by lack, oriented by an unresolved question addressed to the Other, and compelled to negotiate its identity in relation to the desire of others.

In perversion, alienation is present, but separation is short-circuited. The subject is inscribed in the symbolic order yet does not sustain the gap opened by the Other's lack. Instead, it positions itself as the object that completes the Other, thereby neutralizing the question of desire. The division of the subject is not absent but reorganized into a fixed relation to the Other's jouissance.

In psychosis, by contrast, neither alienation nor separation is fully established. Because the Name-of-the-Father is foreclosed, the subject is not properly inscribed in the symbolic order and lacks the structural division that would allow it to take up a position within it. The result is not an absence of experience or intensity but a different configuration in which the Real is no longer symbolically mediated.

Against this background, Fink's claim that "if there is no unconscious, there is no being, no subject, and no desire, strictly speaking" (Fink 1999, 255) can be read more precisely. The point is not that psychotic or perverse subjects are not subjects, but that neurosis, in this sense, most clearly exemplifies a form of subjectivity in which division by lack and the unresolved question of the Other's desire persist.

The neurotic structure contains two principal substructures: hysteria and obsession. Both are organized through repression of symbolic castration and are marked by doubt, yet they articulate the subject's relation to the Other in distinct ways. The hysteric persistently interrogates the desire of the Other and attempts to position itself as the object that would complete it. This positioning does not resolve but sustains the question of the Other's desire. Unlike the pervert, who assumes that this desire can be known and satisfied, the hysteric occupies this position to provoke and keep it open. The focus on sexual identity follows from this: the hysteric seeks to determine what it is for the Other as a sexed being, asking what it means to be desirable as a man or a woman, while eliciting answers it never fully accepts (Lacan 1998 Sem XX, 69–77; Lacan 2006 Écrits, 690).

The obsessional, by contrast, organizes its relation to the Other around the problem of existence and responsibility. Here too doubt is central, but it is managed differently. Rather than asking what it is for the Other, the obsessional asks what it must do to secure its place. The emphasis on action reflects an attempt to stabilize its position through control, yet decisions are repeatedly reconsidered and actions deferred, as if the correct course could be determined in advance. In this way the uncertainty of desire is displaced into the problem of determining what one ought to do and for what one can be held responsible (Lacan 1992 Sem VII, 295–301; Lacan 1998 Sem XI, 235–240).

Beyond Neurosis: Singularity and the Drive

Psychosis, perversion and neurosis are distinct ways of organizing the subject's relation to the loss of jouissance and the impossibility of wholeness introduced by the symbolic order, thereby shaping how it navigates this lack. This raises the question of whether neurosis is the final word.

Although neurosis offers the most stable way of inhabiting the symbolic order, this stability remains tied to the subject's orientation toward the desire of the Other. Lacan's later work suggests another possibility, one that neither escapes lack nor promises reconciliation with a complete self, a complete Other or a final object of satisfaction, but begins where the fantasy of completion is no longer sustained as realizable, even as it continues to structure desire.

What changes is not the structure of desire but the subject's relation to it. The expectation that the Other provides a definitive answer recedes; the Other is no longer approached as its bearer. The relation to the Other remains constitutive, but its function shifts: the question that structures desire no longer directs the subject toward an answer elsewhere but returns it to its own position within that question. As Žižek formulates it, the subject is "thrown into its freedom" precisely where the opacity of the Other's desire can no longer be sustained by fantasy (Žižek 2003, 129).

In this shift, *object a* also changes status. Within neurosis, it remains bound to the fantasy that an object might be found that would finally answer the subject's question and secure its place in the Other's desire. Beyond neurosis, *object a* no longer appears as something that could complete the subject. It comes to mark the structural remainder around which desire and enjoyment circulate. It no longer promises wholeness but indicates the gap that makes such wholeness impossible.

Lacan's later teaching marks a shift from the interplay of the Imaginary and the Symbolic to the Real and the logic of the drive (Lacan 1977 161–200; Lacan 2006, 681–702). What comes into view is the possibility that the subject is no longer defined primarily by its attempt to decipher the desire of the Other. As long as the subject remains a subject of desire, it is caught in a circuit in which the Law forbids, desire transgresses, and the object of fulfillment is endlessly pursued without ever being attained. Desire thus remains tethered to the Other, since it takes shape as a response to what the Other is presumed to want.

The drive follows a different logic. It does not aim at recovering a lost object that would restore wholeness. Instead, it circulates around the structural remainder itself, around *object a*. In doing so, it opens another relation to lack and enjoyment. The subject no longer organizes its position around the search for an object that might answer the question of its desire, but begins to inhabit the very division that structures it. Completion is no longer pursued as a realizable goal but recognized as structurally impossible.

In this configuration, desire remains reactive and dependent on the Law it attempts to exceed, with enjoyment pursued through transgression while recognition continues to be sought from the Other. When enjoyment becomes organized through the drive, this reactive dynamic loosens. As Fink observes, "desire learns how to keep its mouth shut and let enjoyment prevail" (Fink 1997, 211). Desire no longer insists on translating every experience into the question of what the Other wants or into the search for an object that might resolve that question. Instead, enjoyment follows the circuit of the drive.

What Fink describes here is the subject's appropriation of the drives. The drives are no longer experienced simply as pressures imposed by the Other but gradually become something the subject assumes as its own mode of relating to enjoyment. Here the subject sustains its position without resolution and no longer organizes its relation to enjoyment around the search for an answer that could be secured at all.

This position should not be understood as a higher stage, a cure or a form of autonomy in the sense of self-mastery. Nothing in this movement abolishes division or eliminates lack. It designates a different way of inhabiting this condition: an increased capacity to assume and sustain the constitutive incompleteness of subjectivity. What is at stake is not the overcoming of lack but the possibility of relating to it without foreclosure, disavowal or repression as organizing principles.

What Do You Want?

The preceding discussion makes clear that psychosis, perversion, neurosis and beyond are not deviations from a norm but structural positions through which subjects relate to their constitutive lack. Freud already unsettles any strict opposition between the normal and the pathological by showing that the mechanisms underlying symptoms operate throughout ordinary life, to the point that "we are all ill" in a structural sense (Freud 1981, 3418). Lacan radicalizes this insight: these structures are not pathologies opposed to normality but "figures of the normal structure" (Lacan Sem IX, 1962, session 13).

Yet this structural equivalence does not imply that all positions are lived in the same way. What distinguishes them is how the relation to lack is inscribed, sustained and lived, and thus the extent to which it becomes livable. Psychosis is structurally unstable, as symbolic mediation collapses and the subject is exposed to the intrusive presence of the Other. Perversion remains fragile because the lack in the Other is disavowed and must be continuously staged through the organization of law and enjoyment. Neurosis offers a more stable configuration insofar as the subject acknowledges the lack in the Other and situates itself within the symbolic order through it. Singularity implies a different mode of stability: not secured either by symbolic consistency or by the promise of resolution but sustained as an ongoing engagement with lack that remains dynamic and constitutively unsettled.

This marks a shift in the analysis. Without reintroducing a moral distinction between normal and pathological, the structures can be differentiated in terms of how the relation to lack is rendered livable. This, in turn, depends on how the subject situates itself in relation to the question of the Other.

If desire is mediated by the Other, the subject's orientation takes shape through the assumption that the Other knows what is to be desired. The subject addresses the Other as if it possessed the answer, thereby securing orientation while covering over the lack in the Other itself. It is at this point that Lacan formulates the question "Che vuoi?" – "What do you want?" (Lacan 2017, Sem V, 3), not as a request for information but as the structural question through which this relation to lack is organized.

This question can take different forms. Most commonly, it appears as "What do you want from me?", expressing the subject's attempt to locate itself within the field of the Other's desire. Yet insofar as the subject recognizes that the Other does not provide a final answer, the question may return to the subject itself: "What do I want?" This return is not guaranteed, but it marks a shift in position. The Other is no longer approached as the bearer of a final answer but as itself marked by lack; there is no Other of the Other (Lacan 2006, 819).

To assume one's desire is therefore not to step outside the relation to the Other but to remain within it differently. The subject is no longer subordinated to the Other as the locus of an answer, yet cannot step outside it either. What is required is to sustain this tension: the Other does not fully know, yet remains constitutive. Desire is thus not resolved but maintained as a question that cannot be closed.

Seen in this light, the clinical structures can be read as different ways of organizing this question. Some displace or close it through fantasies of certainty, while others sustain it and assume the lack it reveals. What is at stake is the extent to which the subject remains within the question of its own desire without prematurely resolving it. The question is therefore not only how lack and the "Che vuoi?" question are taken up within a given structure but also how these relations compare in terms of livability, including the possibility of regression as well as movement toward a more bearable structural configuration.

At this point, contemporary technological environments intervene in a structurally novel way. Data-driven and algorithmic systems increasingly present themselves as if they could occupy the place of the Other that knows: anticipating preferences and feeding back recommendations that seem to articulate what the subject "really" wants. The question of desire is thereby preempted: instead of confronting an opaque Other, the subject encounters an apparently legible one, and is met with outputs that answer on its behalf, short-circuiting the movement through which it is returned to its own question.

At the same time, this displacement may open a space for reflexive distance. By rendering patterns of preference visible and repeatable, these systems can confront the subject with the mediated character of its own desire, unsettling the assumption that it can be fully known or captured. In doing so, they may not only preempt the question of desire but also return it in a new form, making it possible to take up the question "What do I want?" within and through the very systems that seem to anticipate it.

The following chapter examines this ambivalence, showing how algorithmic environments both simulate a knowing Other and expose its structural lack, producing a double bind in how desire is taken up.

4 Algorithmic Environments and the Displacement of the Symbolic

Algorithmic environments transform the symbolic coordinates through which subjects articulate desire and identify themselves. As these coordinates become increasingly mediated by data-driven, algorithmic, and AI-based systems, the question can no longer be reduced to how technologies influence behavior, but rather how they reorganize the symbolic coordinates through which subjects are addressed and recognized.

This chapter argues that algorithmic environments displace the Symbolic in ways that generate new promises of coherence and wholeness while simultaneously destabilizing the structures through which subjects relate both to the Other and their own lack, thereby making singular subject formation possible.

The chapter proceeds in three steps. First, it shows how algorithmic infrastructures operate as environments that classify and address subjects through data-driven feedback loops. Second, it examines how these environments reshape identification by shifting recognition from symbolic inscription to probabilistic classification, thereby destabilizing its traditional anchors. Third, it analyzes how this displacement reshapes desire, both capturing it and opening the possibility of singular self-formation.

Algorithmic Environments and the Structuring of the Subject

Algorithmic environments cannot be reduced to systems that process information or support decision-making. They reorganize the environments within which subjects encounter others and themselves. What is transformed is not only how actions are guided but the conditions under which subjects are addressed, recognized and come to understand what they want.

Several scholars have attempted to capture this shift from traditional technological infrastructures to what are often described as "smart" or "active" environments (Aydin et al. 2019). De Mul (2015), for example,

DOI: 10.4324/9781042010912-4

introduces the notion of "database identity" to describe how personal and cultural identities in the twenty-first century are increasingly shaped through processes of datafication. Through the digitalization of production processes, financial transactions, GPS signals, surveillance cameras, biometric measurements, smartphones and other connected devices, vast quantities of behavioral traces are continuously captured and processed. As a result, "almost everything becomes part of a global database that will transform how we live, work, and think" (De Mul 2015, 107; see also De Mul 2004). Within such infrastructures, technologies are no longer easily externalized as neutral tools. Instead, they become embedded in the environments through which individuals navigate everyday life (Van Dijck 2014).

The significance of these infrastructures lies not only in the scale of data collection but in the specific way they operate. This operational logic unfolds along three closely related dimensions that together reshape how subjects are positioned and recognized within these environments (Aydin and Possati 2025).

First, data mining operates through processes of categorization and profiling. Individuals and their actions are continuously translated into data and classified within statistical categories derived from large datasets (Cheney-Lippold 2017; Stephens-Davidowitz 2017; Pasquinelli 2023). Instead of addressing users as singular individuals, algorithmic systems position them within predictive groupings such as people with similar preferences, habits or behavioral patterns. In this way, everyday activities such as clicks, searches, purchases or swipes are transformed into profiles that guide how users are subsequently addressed within the system.

Second, these classifications do not operate through fixed meanings but through a connectionist logic in which what matters are the statistical relations between data points. Systems detect patterns across large numbers of interactions and use these patterns to determine what is relevant or likely to occur next. Information that fits recognizable patterns becomes visible and actionable, while what cannot be incorporated into such relations tends to disappear as noise (Malaspina 2018; Sands and Ratey 2023). For users, this means that what becomes visible, relevant or actionable within these environments is increasingly organized through statistical correlations rather than through explicit meanings, intentions or narratives.

Third, these relational structures are continuously recalibrated through feedback loops between user behavior and system adjustment. User interactions generate new data that refine the system's predictive models, while these models in turn influence which options users encounter next. Each click, swipe or selection therefore contributes to reshaping the environment itself. Through this recursive dynamic, algorithmic environments gradually reorganize the pathways through which individuals navigate digital spaces.

Taken together, these characteristics transform technological systems into environments that actively organize how users encounter others and relate to themselves. Rather than merely supporting decisions, these infrastructures structure the field within which decisions become possible by shaping what becomes visible, relevant and actionable through mechanisms such as ranking, filtering and recommendation. What appears to users as an open space of possibilities is therefore already partially structured by algorithmic selection. In this sense, users do not simply act within these environments but are addressed, categorized and guided within them.

Algorithmic environments can be found across many domains of contemporary life, including social media platforms, recommendation systems, online marketplaces and digital dating applications. What these infrastructures share is a common operational logic: they structure interactions through ranking, filtering and prediction.

Digital dating platforms such as Tinder provide a paradigmatic illustration of how such environments operate. Through mechanisms such as ranking systems, matching procedures and interface design, complex social encounters are translated into rapid gestures of selection. The swipe interface, for instance, allows users to evaluate large numbers of profiles within seconds, dramatically reducing friction in the process of interaction while encouraging continuous engagement. What appears as spontaneous discovery or serendipity is therefore mediated by algorithmic curation.

At the same time, machine learning techniques enable these systems to continuously learn from user behavior. Every interaction – clicks, swipes, messages or searches – generates new data that refine the system's predictive models. These models detect not only explicit preferences, such as age or location, but also implicit patterns, including which profiles users linger on or which characteristics recur among successful matches (Noble 2018). In this way, algorithmic environments become increasingly responsive to behavioral traces.

Yet responsiveness should not be mistaken for passivity. Algorithmic infrastructures do not simply reflect user preferences; they actively shape them. By determining which options become visible and how they are presented, these systems guide attention and influence patterns of engagement. User behavior informs algorithmic adjustments, which in turn shape subsequent user behavior. Through this feedback loop, algorithmic environments become dynamic and personalized systems that appear to anticipate and "understand" the user's desires.

One consequence of this dynamic is the emergence of what scholars have described as the "data self." Rather than representing a person as a coherent subject, algorithmic systems construct statistical profiles from patterns extracted from behavioral traces (Cheney-Lippold 2017, 192; Zuboff 2019). These profiles do not simply record past actions; they function as predictive models that anticipate future behavior and influence how individuals are subsequently addressed by the system.

This logic becomes particularly visible in the notion of the digital twin. A digital twin functions as a computational model that simulates aspects of an individual's behavior based on accumulated data (Floridi 2021). Although derived from the user's interactions, this digital double exists independently of the individual and operates within a broader network of models that continuously inform algorithmic predictions. Each digital twin thus becomes part of a larger data ecosystem in which individual behavioral traces contribute to the ongoing adjustment of the system as a whole.

Algorithmic environments produce representations of the self that circulate independently of the subjects who generated them. These representations do not simply describe individuals; they increasingly participate in structuring the environments through which individuals interact with others and relate to themselves. As a result, algorithmic infrastructures not only reshape technological environments but also reorganize the symbolic coordinates through which subjects are addressed, categorized and recognized. In other words, they transform the conditions under which symbolic identification takes place. The next section therefore examines how these technological environments interact with the symbolic processes through which subjects come to identify themselves.

Subject Formation in Algorithmic Environments

Identification and Recognition

If algorithmic infrastructures reorganize the symbolic coordinates through which subjects are addressed and recognized, this transformation directly affects how subjects come to identify themselves. This shift concerns the conditions under which subjects articulate desire and form a sense of self. This requires revisiting Lacan's account of symbolic identification and the role of the Symbolic order in subject formation.

For Lacan, the subject is constituted through its social and symbolic environment. The subject is the result of a symbolic process that involves language, laws and customs (see Zwart 2015, 2017, 2022, 2023; Aydin 2021). Subjectivity emerges through processes of identification that always involve exposure to otherness. This means that there is not first a formed subject that subsequently interacts with its environment (Žižek 2006; Evans 1996, 195–197). Rather, the subject is constituted within what Zwart calls a "symbolic ecosystem" (Zwart 2023, 39): a network of linguistic structures, social expectations and institutional practices that provide individuals with positions through which they can recognize themselves and others. In this sense, the subject is not simply an autonomous individual but first and foremost a being "subjected" to symbolic structures.

At the same time, Lacan insists that identification cannot be reduced to mere subjection. The symbolic order is paradoxical. It is both the condition that makes self-formation possible and the structure that limits it. By providing language, norms and symbolic positions, it enables individuals to situate themselves within a shared social world. Yet these same structures also risk absorbing individuals into preexisting roles and identities. Processes of self-formation therefore unfold within a tension between possibility and constraint: the symbolic order enables identification while simultaneously threatening to reduce the subject to established patterns of recognition.

This paradox becomes clearer when symbolic identification is unpacked into its operative dimensions. Lacan describes several dimensions of this process. The first dimension concerns *numerical identity*. At the most basic level, symbolic identification begins with the simple act of marking a difference. A signifier separates what is marked from what is not marked, thereby creating positions within a symbolic sequence. Through the repeated use of such distinctions, individuals come to occupy a specific place within an ordered series. In this sense, identity initially arises not through substantive meaning or personal qualities but through positional difference. One becomes identifiable simply by being distinguishable from others within a symbolic structure. The subject thus first appears as a countable unit within a symbolic series and experiences itself in two related ways: as a subject that is counted within an order and as a subject capable of counting and distinguishing others within that order. This distinction between being counted and counting becomes crucial when examining how algorithmic systems position individuals within statistical classifications.

The second dimension concerns *nominal identity*. Shortly after birth, individuals are repeatedly addressed through a proper name. Being called by the same name across different situations establishes a stable point of reference through which the subject becomes recognizable to others and to itself (Mooij 2018, 141). The proper name functions as what Lacan calls a unary trait: an empty signifier that marks a subject's position within the symbolic order. Through this process, identity is no longer merely numerical but becomes tied to a symbolic designation that situates the subject within a linguistic and social field. Naming therefore anchors the subject within a network of social relations in which recognition is mediated through language and shared symbolic conventions.

A third dimension concerns *normative identity*: that is, identification with collective ideals, social roles and cultural expectations structured through the expectations of the Other. Names link individuals to families, communities and traditions that project certain aspirations and norms onto the subject. Expectations such as "Jacob will become a great soccer player, just like his father" or "in this community we value solidarity and responsibility" illustrate how individuals are gradually positioned within broader symbolic frameworks. These forms of identification are often expressed through what Lacan calls *insignia* (Lacan 2006, 669): symbols, rituals and practices that mark belonging within particular groups. Initially empty markers of distinction, these signifiers gradually acquire normative meaning and become integrated into the subject's sense of identity.

Taken together, these dimensions illustrate how symbolic identification situates individuals within a structured social order. Through processes of differentiation, naming and identification with shared ideals, subjects acquire a place within the symbolic networks that organize recognition, authority and social belonging. At the same time, these processes do not merely constrain individuals. They also create the conditions under which subjects can orient themselves, negotiate expectations and articulate their own position within the social field. Symbolic identification thus both structures and constrains the subject's position within the field of the Other while at the same time providing the coordinates through which it can assume its place, negotiate its relation to desire and open a space for forms of separation that may take on a more emancipatory thrust.

From this perspective, symbolic identification arises not from an inner psychological core but from a chain of signifiers embedded in social practices, institutions and cultural traditions. The dimensions discussed above – numerical identity, nominal identity and normative identity – illustrate how subjects gradually acquire a place within a symbolic network of distinctions, names and shared ideals. Through these mechanisms, individuals become recognizable within a structured social order and learn to interpret both themselves and others within a shared symbolic horizon. In this sense, the symbolic order stabilizes the more fluid identifications of the Imaginary by introducing rules, norms and expectations that organize social life (Aydin 2021, 216).

Yet the limits of symbolic identification mark the point at which the subject cannot be fully absorbed by the symbolic order. However powerful these structures of differentiation, naming and social recognition may be, they never succeed in fully capturing the subject. Beyond the shaping influence of language and social norms lies the register of the Real. The Real refers to those dimensions of experience that resist symbolization and cannot be fully captured within linguistic or social frameworks. The Real does not precede the symbolic in a chronological sense but emerges precisely through the limitations of symbolic structures themselves. Social norms and symbolic laws evoke the possibility of transgressing them and thereby reveal the structural gap within the symbolic order.

It is precisely this gap that allows for the possibility of singularity. As Aydin notes, "it is by virtue of the Real that an individual cannot be completely absorbed by the general" (Aydin 2021, 217). What escapes generalization and cannot be fully articulated within language often becomes the site of singular self formation (Aydin 2021, 217–218). The Real therefore introduces a dimension of contingency and disruption into processes of identification. It marks the point at which the symbolic order fails to fully capture the subject, opening the possibility that the subject may relate to symbolic structures in unexpected or transformative ways.

Understanding this dynamic is crucial for the analysis that follows. If symbolic identification depends on structures of differentiation, naming and social recognition, the emergence of algorithmic environments raises the question whether these processes are extended or transformed under algorithmic conditions. The next section therefore examines how algorithmic environments interact with these processes of symbolic identification.

Continuity and Disruption

The emergence of algorithmic infrastructures raises a central question: Do data-driven technological environments extend existing processes of symbolic identification, or do they transform the conditions under which subjects articulate their desire and form a sense of self? If symbolic identification unfolds through structures of differentiation, naming and social normativity, how do algorithmic infrastructures intervene in these mechanisms?

Several interpretations have emerged within contemporary Lacanian analyses of digital culture. One influential line of interpretation maintains that algorithmic infrastructures can largely be integrated into the existing Symbolic order without fundamentally disrupting it. From this perspective, Lacan's three registers function as structural coordinates that remain largely invariant even as historical environments change. Technological infrastructures may reshape the context in which identification unfolds, but they do not fundamentally alter its underlying logic. The Symbolic order continues to function as it always has: organizing social life, producing lack and sustaining desire (see, e.g., Zwart 2023; Matviyenko 2015).

Within this framework, algorithmic platforms such as digital dating applications are interpreted as technological extensions of familiar social dynamics. Seeking a partner through a digital platform is not fundamentally different from doing so in offline environments. Individuals continue to pursue recognition, validation and intimacy, and the range of subjective responses remains comparable: some seek affirmation, some idealize partners, others remain uncertain whether they have chosen correctly. What changes is primarily the scale and accessibility of the interactional field. Digital infrastructures enlarge the social playing field, allowing individuals to encounter people they might never meet otherwise. Yet the underlying dynamics of desire and identification remain largely continuous with those found outside digital environments.

A second, more critical line of interpretation shifts the emphasis from continuity to intensification. From this perspective, contemporary digital infrastructures do not fundamentally transform the Symbolic order but significantly amplify dynamics that are already central to capitalist societies. Technology becomes a powerful instrument through which capitalism mobilizes, organizes and exploits desire (Žižek 1997). Data-driven profiling, recommendation systems and predictive analytics contribute to environments in which individuals are constantly encouraged to optimize themselves, pursue recognition and imagine ever more ambitious forms of self-improvement. What is intensified, on this account, are the symbolic mechanisms through which capitalist societies already organize desire: the continuous comparison with others, the pursuit of recognition and success, and the promise that fulfillment lies just beyond the next achievement, acquisition or encounter. Narratives surrounding technological entrepreneurship reinforce this horizon. Figures such as Elon Musk or Bill Gates function as cultural icons of a world in which technological innovation and personal success appear increasingly attainable. In this view, technological environments do not fundamentally transform symbolic identification, but rather intensify its existing horizon: individuals appear unique and self-determining while ultimately pursuing the same fantasy of success, accumulation and self-optimization (Zuboff 2019; see also McGowan 2016).

Digital dating platforms illustrate how such dynamics operate. Through interface design, ranking mechanisms, and tiered subscription models, these platforms structure interactions in ways that sustain continuous engagement. The suggestion that a better match may always be one swipe away keeps desire in motion while preventing closure. In this sense the platform follows a logic familiar from capitalist consumption more broadly: desire is continuously stimulated while fulfillment remains postponed (McGowan 2016). Interactions often become organized around rapid visual evaluation, cycles of validation and competitive comparison, reinforcing dynamics associated with imaginary identification such as objectification and rivalry.

These two interpretations differ in emphasis but ultimately share an important assumption: they both treat algorithmic infrastructures as developments that remain largely continuous with existing symbolic dynamics. A third line of interpretation, however, suggests that contemporary technological environments transform the structure of symbolic mediation itself. From this perspective, the question is no longer simply whether technology extends or intensifies existing symbolic processes but whether it begins to reorganize the mechanisms through which subjects are addressed, recognized and positioned within the Symbolic order.

Lacan's later reflections on technology provide an important starting point for such an interpretation. In Seminar XVII, Lacan explores how modern scientific knowledge increasingly produces objects that intervene directly in the circuits of desire (Lacan 2007 Sem XVII). He introduces the notion of the *alèthosphère*, a technological sphere populated by objects generated through scientific discourse. Within this sphere, technological artifacts, what Lacan calls *lathouses*, function as products of knowledge that circulate within everyday life and address subjects directly. Unlike traditional symbolic mediations, which structure desire through language, law and institutional authority, these objects operate closer to the level of enjoyment itself: they stimulate, capture and redirect desire in ways that are less dependent on established symbolic frameworks (see Loose 2023). This provides a framework for understanding how contemporary algorithmic environments intervene in symbolic mediation.

From this perspective, technological environments may begin to disrupt symbolic mediation in at least two related but distinct ways. First, technological objects increasingly intervene directly in the circuits of desire. They address subjects without passing through many of the slower institutional mediations that traditionally structured how desire was articulated and recognized. Rather than encountering desire primarily through symbolic institutions such as family, education, religion or cultural traditions, subjects increasingly encounter technological objects that promise immediate forms of satisfaction, optimization or recognition. In Lacanian terms, desire becomes increasingly engaged by objects that appear to offer direct responses to the subject's longing, thereby partially bypassing the symbolic processes through which desire was historically mediated.

Second, algorithmic infrastructures transform the way subjects themselves are identified and addressed. Instead of being positioned primarily through symbolic recognition grounded in names, roles and institutional frameworks, individuals are increasingly categorized through statistical correlations and predictive models. Rather than deriving legitimacy from shared norms, traditions or linguistic recognition, these systems operate through calculation, pattern detection and automated decision processes. As a result, the mechanisms through which subjects are addressed gradually shift from symbolic recognition toward forms of algorithmic classification that position individuals within probabilistic categories rather than stable symbolic identities.

Feminist analyses of digital platforms have also drawn attention to transformations in regimes of visibility, evaluation and recognition within digitally mediated environments (Illouz 2007; Gill 2007; Banet-Weiser 2018). Rather than merely intensifying existing dynamics of desire, these studies suggest that platform architectures reorganize the conditions under which subjects appear, are evaluated and become recognizable to others. Algorithmic infrastructures therefore participate not only in the circulation of desire but also in reshaping the symbolic frameworks through which recognition and identification occur.

Several contemporary Lacanian theorists have developed related insights in analyses of digital culture. Tomšič (2015) suggests that contemporary technological infrastructures generate new forms of ideological interpellation that reshape the subject's relation to knowledge, enjoyment and power. More recently, scholars such as Matthew Flisfeder (2021), Bandinelli and Johanssen (2022) and Rambatan and Johanssen (2021) have examined how algorithmic platforms organize visibility, fantasy and enjoyment within digitally mediated environments (see also Bown 2015). Their analyses demonstrate how algorithmic infrastructures increasingly participate in structuring the circuits of desire through which subjects encounter others and themselves.

Building on these contributions, the analysis developed here shifts the focus in two ways. First, rather than concentrating primarily on specific platforms or on the dynamics of enjoyment, this study examines how algorithmic environments more broadly reorganize the symbolic coordinates through which subjects are recognized, positioned and oriented in relation to their desire. Second, the analysis connects these transformations of symbolic mediation to the central question that runs throughout this book: how technological environments reshape the conditions under which processes of de-identification and singular self-formation become possible.

In conventional symbolic environments, subjects become recognizable through symbolic inscription. Names, roles and institutional frameworks situate individuals within relatively stable coordinates that define who they are and how they relate to others. In algorithmic environments, by contrast, individuals increasingly become legible through data-driven correlations that classify and rank and predict behavior. Recognition becomes less dependent on symbolic naming and institutional positioning and more on computational classification. Individuals are addressed less as symbolically recognized identities and more as data profiles that can be sorted, evaluated and predicted. This displacement raises the question of how profoundly contemporary technological environments unsettle established forms of symbolic identification.

De-Identification

The previous section introduced a third line of interpretation according to which contemporary technological infrastructures transform the structure of symbolic mediation itself. If this is the case, algorithmic environments do not merely extend or intensify existing dynamics of symbolic identification. They also interfere with the mechanisms through which subjects are traditionally recognized, positioned and oriented within the Symbolic order.

To understand this transformation more concretely, we must examine how algorithmic infrastructures interact with different forms of symbolic identification. Earlier, numerical identity, nominal identity and normative identity were discussed as ways in which subjects become positioned within symbolic structures: through differentiation within an ordered sequence, through inscription by a proper name and through identification with ideals. These forms are not simply replaced by algorithmic systems. Rather, they are reworked in ways that loosen their symbolic anchoring and introduce new modes of classification, profiling and feedback (Aydin and Possati 2025).

The first transformation concerns *numerical identity*. In Lacanian terms, the subject emerges through differentiation. It becomes one among others, positioned within a symbolic sequence and able to distinguish itself from other positions within that order. Numerical identity therefore depends not merely on being counted but on being situated within a structured field of symbolic distinctions.

Algorithmic classification changes this dynamic. Instead of assigning subjects a relatively stable position within a symbolic sequence, algorithmic systems classify individuals through probabilistic correlations derived from large datasets. The subject appears less as someone occupying a determinate symbolic place, such as a family role, professional position or social status, and more as a shifting cluster of behavioral probabilities. It is identified as someone likely to watch certain films, buy certain products, respond to certain prompts or interact with certain profiles. The subject is now primarily distinguished not by its place within an ordered symbolic structure but by patterns inferred from aggregated behavioral traces.

This also affects the subject's position as the one who counts and distinguishes. Agorithmic systems process relations at a scale and level of complexity that exceed ordinary symbolic comprehension. The subject is still counted, but it no longer fully participates in the symbolic ordering through which that counting becomes intelligible. Numerical identity is therefore not abolished but reorganized: symbolic differentiation is increasingly supplemented by statistical classification.

The second transformation concerns *nominal identity*. Within the Symbolic, the proper name anchors the subject within a linguistic, social and institutional framework. A name is not merely a label. It links the subject to family relations, legal recognition, biographical continuity and institutional inscription. A passport, for instance, connects a name to a date of birth, nationality and recognized civic identity. In this way, nominal identity secures a relatively durable relation between the subject and the symbolic order.

In algorithmic environments, this anchoring function becomes less decisive. Identification increasingly takes place through profiles generated from behavioral data rather than through institutionally secured names. The individual appears not primarily as a named subject but as a variable within a dataset, connected to other variables through inferred correlations. Recommendation systems, targeted advertising, risk scores and predictive analytics do not need to know who the subject is in a symbolic or biographical sense. They need to know how this profile behaves, to which patterns it belongs and what it is likely to do next. Nominal identity is therefore supplemented, and sometimes displaced, by dynamic profiling. The name remains, but it is no longer the privileged anchor of identification.

The third transformation concerns *normative identity*. In Lacanian theory, the subject encounters images, expectations and ideals that promise coherence, recognition and future possibility. These ideals may be projected by parents, institutions, cultural authorities or broader social norms. They orient the subject, but they also remain at a distance. The subject can identify with them, strive toward them and internalize them but never fully coincide with them. This distance is crucial because it sustains desire.

Algorithmic profiling operates according to a different logic. It does not primarily present the subject with an external ideal of what it might become. It returns predictions based on what the subject, or similar subjects, have done before. A recommendation system does not say: this is what you ought to become. It says, more quietly and effectively: this is what you are likely to want, choose, watch, buy or desire next. The subject is therefore confronted not with an aspirational ideal that must be negotiated and internalized but with a behavioral reflection derived from its own traces.

To highlight the subtle but crucial shift, two consequences can be identified. First, the distance between subject and ideal is reduced. In symbolic identification, the ideal comes from elsewhere: from the Other, from institutions, from cultural expectations, from images of what one might become. Algorithmic feedback, by contrast, often appears as a mirror of the subject's own behavior. It confronts the subject not with an external image of possibility but with a predictive version of itself.

Second, these profiles are not normative ideals in the strong sense. They do not articulate what is admirable, meaningful or socially desirable. They register statistical regularities and translate them into likely next steps. Normative orientation is therefore supplemented by predictive feedback.

Once the distance between subject and ideal is reduced and normative orientation is displaced by predictive feedback, the structure of recognition itself is transformed. In Lacan's theory of subject formation, recognition is mediated by the desire of the Other. Individuals seek validation from parents, peers and institutions whose recognition shapes their sense of self.

Algorithmic environments do not eliminate recognition but reorganize it. Users receive encouragement from applications such as Duolingo, emotional responses from conversational agents such as Replika, and validation through likes and comments on platforms such as YouTube or Instagram. Recognition persists, but its structure shifts. The identity of the

Other behind these interactions often remains ambiguous: online communities may consist of anonymous users, automated systems or hybrid configurations in which motivations and agencies are unclear. The symbolic authority of the Other thus becomes more diffuse and fragmented.

Some critical interpretations build on this development and suggest that such transformations may foster regressive psychological dynamics in which subjects become increasingly immersed in cycles of feedback and validation (Paranjpe 2022; Kemberg 2020). If algorithmic environments transform how recognition is organized, they also alter how subjects relate to the Other whose recognition structures their sense of self. Rather than supporting reflective forms of identification mediated by relatively stable symbolic authorities, these environments tend to privilege more immediate responses oriented toward visibility, affirmation and continuous engagement. Recognition does not disappear but increasingly unfolds through algorithmically mediated responses whose source and authority remain opaque.

Taken together, these developments illustrate how algorithmic environments reorganize established forms of symbolic identification. Numerical positioning within symbolic sequences is increasingly supplemented by probabilistic classification, symbolic naming by algorithmic profiling, and aspirational ideals by predictive models derived from behavioral traces. Yet these transformations do not amount to a simple erosion of symbolic structure.

Algorithmic infrastructures introduce new classificatory frameworks through which subjects are sorted, predicted and addressed. What emerges is not a straightforward breakdown of the symbolic order but a more complex dynamic in which disruption and reproduction occur simultaneously. Established symbolic anchors loosen, while new systems of categorization and recognition take shape that organize how individuals appear within algorithmic environments.

This dual movement can be understood as a process of symbolic de-identification. The symbolic anchors through which subjects have traditionally been recognized and positioned lose part of their stabilizing force. This may open space for a less rigid relation to inherited identities and for experimentation with alternative forms of identification. At the same time, algorithmic infrastructures do not dissolve structures of identification. They rearticulate them through new forms of classification, prediction and feedback, which increasingly mediate how subjects understand themselves and others.

Understanding this ambivalence is crucial for the argument that follows. If algorithmic environments loosen established symbolic anchors while simultaneously introducing new systems of classification and recognition, they also reshape the conditions under which desire is articulated, directed and sustained. The next section therefore examines how these transformations of symbolic mediation affect the relation between desire and singular self-formation in algorithmic environments.

Desire and Singularity in Algorithmic Environments

Algorithmic environments transform not only how subjects are identified but how desire is oriented and sustained. In Lacanian terms, desire takes shape within symbolic coordinates that indicate what subjects may want, pursue and become. As these coordinates shift, so too does the structure of desire, and with it the conditions under which subjects can form themselves. The question, then, is whether and how singularity may take shape under these conditions, as a form of subject formation not fully determined by given symbolic or algorithmic orientations.

In Lacanian terms, the subject is constituted by lack, and desire emerges from this structural absence that cannot be eliminated but continually propels it beyond what is given (Lolli 2022). Desire expresses this absence while searching for something that might fill it. It unfolds as an open-ended movement in which subjects orient themselves toward objects, ideals and forms of recognition that promise fulfillment. For desire to take direction, however, it requires coordinates that indicate where fulfillment might be sought and what one should strive to become. The effectiveness of such coordinates lies not in actually delivering wholeness but in sustaining the belief that such fulfillment might be achieved.

Across different historical configurations, societies have organized these coordinates in different ways. Roughly speaking, three regimes can be distinguished: classical symbolic orders, late modern and postmodern conditions, and contemporary algorithmic environments. These regimes differ not only in the frameworks that orient desire but also in how subjects experience the source from which expectations, recognition and authority appear to arise.

In classical symbolic orders, desire is oriented through relatively stable institutions and shared frameworks such as religion, tradition and enduring social hierarchies. These provide relatively clear answers to questions about what one should want, how one should live and who one should become. Desire is organized through durable narratives that promise meaning and fulfillment, even though this promise is never fully realized. The locus of the Other remains relatively legible, anchored in recognized authorities and forms of life.

In late modern and postmodern conditions, these frameworks lose much of their stability. The decline of grand narratives does not eliminate the horizon of promise that structures desire but transforms it into more diffuse and secular forms. Ideologies such as socialism, democracy and faith in scientific progress continue to function as residual frameworks, sustaining the belief that collective projects or rational progress may still deliver fulfillment. Under these conditions, subjects orient their desire toward a plurality of competing promises rather than a single symbolic authority.

Algorithmic environments introduce a further transformation. Here the vectors that orient desire are no longer primarily articulated through symbolic discourse or cultural narratives but are increasingly generated through computational processes such as rankings, recommendations, trending metrics and predictive feedback. Desire is not merely exposed to plurality; it is continuously modulated through infrastructures that analyze past behavior and anticipate what one is likely to want next.

Under these conditions, subjects encounter indications of what they should want without a clearly identifiable agent who articulates or authorizes these expectations. Trends, influencers, platform metrics and recommendation systems constantly suggest new objects of desire, yet the authority behind these suggestions remains shifting and opaque. Desire continues to be organized through responses coming from the outside, but the locus from which these expectations emerge becomes diffuse and embedded in technological infrastructures rather than anchored in stable institutions or traditions.

This algorithmic transformation can generate a distinctive form of disorientation. The question that Lacan formulates as *Che vuoi?* – what do you want? – returns to the subject with renewed force. Such moments are rarely neutral. They often appear as disruptive or even traumatic encounters with the limits of symbolic mediation (see also Aydin 2017). When the coordinates that previously organized desire become unstable, subjects may find themselves confronted more directly with the question of their own desire.

Yet this disorientation does not automatically lead to singular self-formation. More often, it provokes attempts to restore orientation. Roughly speaking, three responses can be distinguished.

The first response consists in withdrawing from technological environments and returning to earlier symbolic frameworks. Faced with instability, individuals may seek renewed certainty in traditional authorities, cultural identities or ideological positions that promise stable answers to what one should desire and become. This restores familiar coordinates and prevents subjective disintegration but primarily reinstates given orientations rather than opening space for singular self-formation. Instead, it renews investment in earlier symbolic orders. This analysis does not assess whether withdrawal from algorithmic environments, without a return to such frameworks, may enable singular self-formation outside them.

A second response unfolds within algorithmic environments themselves. Here, subjects attempt to reestablish orientation by adapting to the logic of algorithmic mediation. These responses broadly correspond to the clinical structures discussed earlier: psychosis, perversion and neurosis.

In one form, subjects increasingly identify with the classifications produced by algorithmic systems. They encounter themselves as aggregates of preferences, behavioral tendencies and predicted actions. Repeated exposure to such representations through advertisements, recommendations, and search results can lead to their incorporation into self-understanding. In its most extreme form, this position approaches psychosis: the distinction between subject and classification collapses, and the individual comes to coincide with the categories produced by the system.

A second form resembles the perverse structure. Here, subjects do not simply identify with classifications but adapt themselves to the logic through which systems operate. They learn how profiles, preferences and behavioral signals are processed and adjust their conduct accordingly to obtain favorable responses from platforms and recommendation systems. Algorithmic infrastructures are treated as mechanisms whose rules can be navigated. Yet precisely through this strategic adaptation, the subject increasingly aligns itself with the operational logic of the system and becomes an extension of the very mechanism it seeks to exploit. Desire remains captured within its circuits.

Both tendencies are visible in contemporary consumer culture. On the one hand, algorithmic infrastructures continually recommend products, experiences and identities that correspond to previously recorded preferences. In many cases this produces cycles of largely unquestioned accumulation: overflowing wardrobes, multiple cars, endless gadgets and an abundance of lifestyle accessories. The subject increasingly aligns itself with the classifications and predictions generated by the system, allowing desire to be steered by algorithmic correlations.

On the other hand, users learn to adapt strategically to the logic of these systems. They curate their own data traces, adjusting online profiles, preferences and consumption patterns to obtain more favorable responses from platforms and recommendation systems. Here the subject does not simply coincide with algorithmic classifications but learns how to navigate and exploit them. Yet even in this case, desire remains captured within the circuits generated by the system itself.

Romele (2019) describes this development as the emergence of a digital habitus. In algorithmic environments, individuals increasingly encounter themselves through typified representations generated by data analysis. Over time, these representations may come to function as meaningful descriptions of who one is (Romele 2019, 151–152; see also Grosman and Reigeluth 2019). In some cases, subjects align themselves with these classifications, allowing their desires and choices to be guided by predictions derived from their past behavior. In other cases, they learn to anticipate and accommodate the logic of the system, adjusting their conduct so that the responses generated by algorithmic infrastructures become more favorable. In both cases, desire is organized through predictive correlations that encourage subjects to continue desiring more of what they have already desired.

A third form corresponds to the neurotic structure. Here, subjects remain invested in the promises offered by technological environments but oscillate between belief and disappointment. They repeatedly experience the sense that the desired object has finally been found, only to discover shortly afterward that fulfillment slips away. Algorithmic infrastructures intensify this oscillation by continually presenting new objects, identities and experiences as potential answers to desire.

Technological ecosystems illustrate this dynamic particularly clearly. Consider the ecosystem created by Apple. Its tightly integrated network of devices and services promises coherence, innovation and belonging, encouraging sustained investment. Each new product launch mobilizes anticipation and collective excitement, suggesting that the long-awaited object may finally deliver what was previously missing. Yet almost immediately after its release, attention shifts toward the next anticipated innovation. Desire is thus repeatedly reignited and redirected, sustaining a cycle of expectation and disappointment without resolution.

Across these forms the subject remains captured within the horizon of the algorithmic environment. Rather than dissolving symbolic structures, these environments generate new forms of symbolic normativity that organize expectations, recognition and patterns of behavior. Whether subjects identify with algorithmic classifications, adapt themselves to system logic or continue to pursue the objects it promises, their desire remains structured by the infrastructures that guide and evaluate them.

Yet these responses do not exhaust the possibilities opened by algorithmic environments. Precisely because algorithmic infrastructures destabilize and continuously recalibrate the coordinates that orient desire, they may expose subjects more directly to the question of their own desire. Instead of seeking answers in earlier symbolic orders or in algorithmic classifications, subjects may begin to assume responsibility for this question themselves. In such cases, the instability of technological environments does not simply produce conformity but may open a space in which individuals confront the lack that structures their desire and articulate their own position in relation to it. In Lacanian terms, this marks the point at which the subject may move toward a singular form of subjectivity.

Whether such confrontations lead to singular self-formation or to new forms of subjugation remains an open question. The destabilization of symbolic coordinates does not in itself produce singularity but depends on how subjects respond to the absence of stable answers to the question of their own desire. The following chapter develops this argument further through a paradigmatic case, using Tinder to examine how desire unfolds within algorithmically organized environments and how subjects are structured within them.

5 Technological Promises and Clinical Structures

Algorithmic environments unsettle the symbolic coordinates that orient desire and confront subjects with shifting indications of what to want. The question is how desire is organized under these conditions. This chapter addresses that question by applying Lacan's clinical structures of psychosis, perversion and neurosis to algorithmically organized environments. Tinder serves as a paradigmatic case because the search for a partner foregrounds desire, recognition and lack in an existentially charged way, rendering the effects of technological mediation especially clear.

The chapter proceeds in two steps. It first examines Tinder as a technological environment in which desire is organized, focusing on the promises that structure it. It then analyzes how subjects position themselves in relation to these dynamics through different clinical configurations, opening the question of whether and how more singular relations to desire become possible.

Tinder as a Paradigmatic Case

Tinder and the Organization of Desire

Tinder presents itself as a technological solution to one of the most fundamental uncertainties of human life: how to find and connect with others in the search for intimacy, companionship or love. Through profiles, photographs and algorithmically curated suggestions, the platform promises to facilitate encounters that might otherwise remain unlikely or impossible. At first glance, Tinder appears simply as a tool that expands the range of potential partners and simplifies the process of meeting them.

Yet Tinder does more than facilitate encounters. The platform organizes and amplifies the dynamics of desire itself. By presenting a continuous stream of potential partners, it suggests that the long-awaited encounter might always be just one swipe away. Each profile appears as a

DOI: 10.4324/9781042010912-5

possible answer to the question of whom one might want, desire or become intimate with.

In Lacanian terms, this dynamic can be understood through the notion of *object a*, the object-cause of desire. Desire is never directed toward a final object capable of resolving the subject's lack. Instead, it organizes through substitutes that momentarily appear to embody what is missing. Tinder structures this dynamic technologically: each profile functions as a placeholder for *object a*, an image that appears to promise the missing element that might complete the subject.

The interface intensifies this dynamic through a simple but powerful mechanism: the swipe. With each movement of the finger, one potential object of desire disappears and another immediately takes its place. Desire is therefore not brought to rest but continuously reactivated. Each new profile appears as a possible answer to the question that the previous one failed to resolve.

Matches further reinforce this process. When two users express mutual interest, the platform signals this through the familiar message, "It's a match." At that moment the possibility emerges that the encounter might finally move from fantasy to reality. Yet even here the promise remains fragile. Conversations may never begin, interactions may quickly fade, or the anticipated encounter may fail to deliver the expected fulfillment. The cycle of anticipation and disappointment therefore continues, prompting the subject to return once more to the endless sequence of profiles.

In this sense, Tinder does not simply mediate desire; it organizes its movement. By continuously presenting new potential objects and structuring the rhythm through which they appear and disappear, the platform technologically amplifies the metonymic character of desire described by Lacan. Each new profile appears as the possible bearer of what is missing, while the impossibility of final satisfaction ensures that desire continues to circulate.

Tinder in Context

In its early years, internet dating was often associated with individuals who struggled to meet partners through conventional social settings. Dating websites, and later applications, were therefore framed as solutions for socially isolated or awkward individuals. Over the past decade, however, online dating has become a mainstream practice. Platforms such as Tinder, Badoo, Bumble, Hinge, OkCupid, Grindr and Brenda have attracted hundreds of millions of users worldwide, promising companionship, pleasure and happiness. Among these, Tinder remains the most prominent and culturally recognizable example, and will therefore serve as the primary case study in this chapter. At the same time, the analysis applies more broadly to contemporary dating platforms and, more generally, to algorithmically mediated environments in which encounters, preferences and desires are increasingly organized through data-driven systems.

Founded in 2012, Tinder allows users to like or reject profiles through a simple swiping mechanism. A conversation becomes possible only when both users express interest, resulting in a match. Profiles typically include photographs, age, distance and a short personal description. The platform has attracted more than 75 million monthly active users across more than 190 countries, is available in 40 languages, and has generated more than 60 billion matches, with approximately 1.6 billion swipes per day and around 1.5 million dates each week. In 2023 alone, Tinder generated approximately $1.91 billion in revenue (Iqbal 2025; Wise 2023). Online dating can therefore no longer be considered a marginal phenomenon. Platforms such as Tinder increasingly shape how people encounter one another, form expectations about intimacy and interpret their own desirability.

Scholars have approached the effects of dating apps on intimacy and relationships from different perspectives. Some argue that such platforms weaken emotional attachment, loyalty and long-term commitment. Eva Illouz offers one of the most influential critical accounts. In works such as *Cold Intimacies* (2007) and *Why Love Hurts* (2012), she argues that dating platforms preserve the cultural ideal of romantic love while transforming the emotional infrastructures through which love is experienced (Illouz and Kotliar 2022). Drawing on Lasch (1979) and Bauman (2000), she suggests that the logic of consumer culture has penetrated intimate life, producing what she describes as capitalist subjectivity (Illouz 2022; see also Illouz 1997). Within this framework, emotions become commodified into what she calls emodities (Illouz 2017), which in technologically mediated environments evolve further into techno emodities (Illouz 2022, 231). The digital architecture of choice (Illouz 2012, 91) encourages short-term encounters and instant gratification. Tinder, in this view, transforms romantic encounters into transactions, contributing to declining emotional investment (Illouz 2012, 53).

Other scholars challenge this interpretation. Empirical studies do not consistently support the claim that dating apps undermine commitment or intimacy. Rosenfeld (2018) shows that most heterosexual adults continue to enter relatively traditional forms of partnership, and that casual sexual relationships remain less widespread than often assumed. Other researchers suggest that contemporary dating practices often reaffirm rather than dissolve traditional norms surrounding love and commitment (Carter 2017; Van Hooff 2013, 2017; Carter 2012; Carter and Duncan 2016; Jamieson 1998; Smart 2007). Rather than undermining love and commitment, modern dating forms, they argue, free relationships from societal restrictions and allow them to be more directly shaped by personal choice.

The aim of this study is not to resolve this empirical debate. While some users report finding lasting relationships and others describe frustration or alienation, the broader consequences of dating apps remain difficult to determine. Instead, the present analysis approaches Tinder as a technological environment that shapes how subjects encounter themselves and others. It functions not as an object of sociological evaluation but as a case through which the relation between technological infrastructures and desire can be examined.

Although this perspective shares with Illouz an interest in how digital platforms mediate intimacy and selfhood, it departs from her framework at a more fundamental level. Illouz situates these transformations within shifts in capitalism, consumer culture and institutional arrangements. The present analysis instead brackets these socioeconomic explanations and focuses on the structure of desire itself. The question is therefore not how platforms reshape relationships at the level of norms or practices but how they reorganize the imaginary and symbolic coordinates that give direction to desire. In doing so, they shape how subjects interpret what they want, recognize themselves in relation to others and orient themselves within possible attachments.

Tinder's Promise

To understand Tinder's promise, it is necessary to consider what the platform explicitly and implicitly promises and to what extent it delivers on that promise. On its homepage (Tinder, accessed February 25, 2026), Tinder initially adopts a light hearted tone: "Single people, listen up: If you're looking for love, want to start dating, or just keep it casual, you need to be on Tinder." Yet a few sentences later the tone shifts toward stronger assurances: "Want to get into a relationship? You got it. Trying to find some new friends? Say no more" (Tinder, accessed February 25, 2026).

The testimonials featured on the homepage are even more explicit: "THANK YOU for making it possible for me to meet my soulmate" (Victoria and Bayleigh); "Thanks to Tinder I have found the love of my life and we are to be married" (Courtney and Miranda); "We both fell hard and fast and knew we had found our person fairly quickly" (Magdalena and Annie). Strikingly, many of these testimonials begin with statements such as "I just wanted to have some fun" or "I didn't expect to meet anyone" but end with affirmations like "Fast forward 9 months, and we had become inseparable," "forever grateful" or "I am married." In these narratives Tinder appears as the technological mediator that finally enables the long-awaited solution.

Of course, such testimonials hardly provide an accurate or representative picture of users' experiences. A very different narrative appears on review platforms. Consider Trustpilot: "Literally the worst online experience I've ever had, terms and conditions are horrendous … avoid this app." Or: "Great site if you like Jabba the Hutt/Cookie Monster lookalikes …

low end of the gene pool." Or simply: "Tbh just go out and meet someone. All apps are a scam and waste of money." Of the 3,517 reviews, 87 percent give Tinder a one-star rating (Trustpilot, accessed February 25, 2026). On Reddit, users express similar disillusionment: "The modern world has commodified everything. The machine will profit from your loneliness." Or: "If my boyfriend and I ever break up, I'm doomed." Or simply: "No, I think I'll stay single. Thanks!" (Reddit, accessed February 25, 2026). On ConsumerAffairs, Tinder scores two out of five stars, with complaints about fake profiles, spam messages and unsuitable matches (ConsumerAffairs, accessed January 7, 2026).

Clearly these observations are anecdotal. It may well be that people with positive experiences are less likely to leave reviews, while dissatisfied users are more inclined to express their frustration online. I do not claim that such testimonials and reviews constitute solid empirical research, let alone that they establish any causal relationship between Tinder use and users' psychological states.

A review of more methodologically robust studies indicates that relatively few establish a clear link between Tinder use and increased happiness or life satisfaction. Her and Timmermans (2020), using an online survey of 296 U.S. adults, argue that Tinder use may have detrimental effects for compulsive users, those seeking romantic partners and individuals prone to social comparison. At the same time, the study suggests that users who approach Tinder more casually, who use the app less intensively or who are relatively successful in securing matches may experience improved well-being. Similarly, Barrada and Castro (2020), in a survey of 1,261 Spanish university students, found either no or only very small differences in emotional well-being between users and nonusers. Erevik et al. (2020), using a survey of 5,253 students in Bergen, Norway, found that Tinder users reported more symptoms of anxiety, were more likely to engage in binge drinking and drug use, and had higher levels of impulsivity. While Tinder users were more likely to enter romantic relationships, the researchers suggest that this was likely due to other variables rather than the app itself.

Another study by Bleize et al. (2023), based on more than 1,000 respondents aged 18–34 in the United States and the United Kingdom, found that users of dating apps reported lower satisfaction with their relationship status than did nonusers. However, it remained unclear whether dating app use caused dissatisfaction or whether dissatisfied individuals were simply more likely to use such apps in the first place.

Sharabi and Dorrance-Hall (2024), surveying 923 married U.S. adults, about half of whom had met their spouse through online dating, found that online daters reported slightly less satisfying and stable marriages, a phenomenon they termed the "online dating effect." A study from Stanford Medicine (Vera Cruz et al. 2023) similarly found that satisfaction with both dating apps and the dates that followed correlated strongly with users' motivations for using them, whether entertainment, distraction, or self-esteem. In particular, participants who used dating apps primarily as a coping mechanism tended to report the lowest levels of satisfaction.

Even on the basis of more reliable research, it remains difficult to draw firm conclusions about whether dating apps such as Tinder are good or bad for users. Too many variables are involved: personality traits, expectations, life context and prior experiences. Not only causal relationships but even correlations remain difficult to establish. Unsurprisingly, most studies therefore call for broader and more systematic research before any definitive conclusions can be reached.

Still, the question of why such apps and platforms are so attractive to users remains, especially given that it is far from clear what users actually gain from them, and that many studies lean more negative than positive. How, then, can we explain the exponential growth in the use of Tinder and similar dating technologies?

One plausible hypothesis is that Tinder's appeal lies not in the guarantee of a successful match or lasting relationship but in the way it radically simplifies the process of seeking a partner. Tinder transforms the search for a partner into a gamified, low-threshold digital experience. One no longer needs to attend weddings, navigate complex social settings or hope for serendipitous encounters at parties. Instead, a few taps suffice: download the app, enter basic information, upload a handful of photos – and one is ready to begin. For those who are anxious, shy or introverted, this lowered threshold makes entry into the dating world significantly less daunting. Even rejection is made easier, reduced to a gesture, a swipe left, stripping it of its usual emotional weight. In this sense, Tinder makes things easier.

Yet what is made easier is not the attainment of a meaningful connection or deep compatibility. What is streamlined is the mechanism of searching itself: the repetitive cycle of looking, swiping and matching. The seduction lies in the frictionless process, not in its outcome. Admittedly, Tinder expands the pool of potential partners considerably, which can create the illusion of increased efficiency or fruitfulness. But whether this ease also improves the likelihood of finding the right partner or leads to what Thaler and Sunstein describe as a longer, healthier, better life is a different matter entirely. It serves as a reminder that making the search easier does not necessarily bring one closer to what one desires. The appeal of platforms such as Tinder therefore cannot be fully explained in terms of ease or behavioral steering alone. What such explanations leave largely untouched is the structure of desire itself and the way technological environments sustain the expectation that the next possibility might finally deliver what previous ones did not.

At the same time, Tinder does not merely organize the search for others; it also exposes users to the question of how they themselves appear to others. Profiles function not only as windows onto potential partners but also as mirrors through which users evaluate their own desirability. In swiping through others, users are simultaneously aware that they themselves are being seen, assessed and potentially desired or rejected. The platform therefore stages not only the desire for another person but also the desire to be desired. Users are not merely searching for someone they might want; they are also seeking confirmation that they themselves are wanted. In this way Tinder situates users simultaneously as subjects who desire and as objects that may be desired by others.

Equally crucial are the expectations that users bring to the platform. A key insight, confirmed by the Stanford study and others, is that users' satisfaction with Tinder depends largely on the motivations they bring to it. Are they seeking distraction, validation, casual encounters, social connection or the elusive partner who might finally resolve feelings of incompleteness? These expectations shape how users relate to the platform and, more fundamentally, how they relate to themselves.

What remains insufficiently explained in these accounts is why subjects remain invested in this cycle, despite its repeated failure to deliver what it promises. At this point the analysis converges with the Lacanian framework developed earlier. What matters is the structure of desire itself and how subjects relate to it. The promise of Tinder therefore resides not in the matches it produces but in the anticipatory horizon it creates: the persistent suggestion that the next encounter might finally deliver what previous ones did not.

Tinder as Tragedy of Desire

Many accounts of Tinder's popularity emphasize convenience, entertainment or the expansion of potential partner pools. These factors undoubtedly play an important role. Yet they do not fully explain why subjects remain so receptive to technological promises in a domain marked by particularly strong expectations and uncertainties: the search for a partner. What is at stake, therefore, is not simply the effectiveness of the platform but the structure of desire that renders its promise compelling.

Users who approach Tinder for entertainment or distraction often report fewer disappointments than those who hope to find a partner who will finally complete them. Expectations clearly shape the experience of the platform. Yet this difference cannot be explained solely in psychological terms as a matter of more or less realistic expectations. For Lacan, the difficulty lies deeper, in the structure of desire itself. Desire is organized around a constitutive lack that no object can ultimately fill. When a partner is invested with the hope of resolving this lack, the relationship becomes burdened with a promise that cannot be fulfilled.

This dynamic becomes especially visible in intimate relationships. Many objects can temporarily function as substitutes for what Lacan calls the object-cause of desire: *object a*. Yet relationships tend to carry far greater expectations. For many, choosing a partner shapes the horizon of everyday life: shared projects, identities, roles and futures become organized around that choice. In this sense a relationship forms a micro symbolic order that structures recognition and belonging. When a partner becomes unconsciously invested with the role of *object a*, the relationship becomes organized through fantasy: the partner appears as the figure through which the subject imagines that its lack might finally be resolved.

Tinder intensifies precisely this investment by staging the partner as a selectable object within a continuous stream of possibilities. Seen in this light, the attraction of dating platforms becomes easier to understand. Tinder does not simply facilitate encounters between individuals; it organizes the search for a partner within a technological environment that appears to make the discovery of the "right" partner increasingly manageable. Through profiles, matches and algorithmic filtering the platform suggests that the uncertainty surrounding desire can be reduced.

Rather than fulfilling desire, however, platforms such as Tinder reorganize the conditions under which desire continues to circulate. By presenting an apparently endless sequence of potential partners, the platform sustains the expectation that the object capable of resolving desire might still be encountered. Each new profile appears as a possible embodiment of what is missing, renewing the movement of desire rather than bringing it to rest.

In this respect, Tinder makes visible a broader dynamic characteristic of contemporary technological environments. Many data-driven systems promise orientation in situations of fundamental uncertainty by transforming complex questions into navigable sequences of choices. Whether recommending products, careers or partners, algorithmic infrastructures present themselves as tools for optimizing selection.

From a Lacanian perspective, however, the fundamental problem cannot be resolved at the level of choice. The difficulty lies not in the abundance of options but in the structure of subjectivity itself. The subject is constitutively split, and full jouissance is structurally impossible. No object, no matter how carefully selected, can finally coincide with the object a that animates desire. Technological systems therefore reorganize how subjects encounter this structural impossibility.

The way subjects respond to this split has a tragic structure. A classical image of tragedy helps illuminate this dynamic. In Sophocles' Oedipus Rex, the attempt to escape a prophecy becomes the mechanism through which it is fulfilled (Sophocles 1984). Oedipus flees in order to avoid his fate, yet through this very attempt he realizes it. The tragedy lies not simply in inevitability but in the fact that the effort to avoid the outcome produces it. This is not merely an illustrative parallel; it expresses the same structural logic.

A similar paradox characterizes the structure of desire. Desire is organized around a constitutive lack that cannot be eliminated. In pursuing objects, the subject seeks what Lacan calls the lost *object a*. Yet each object obtained merely reactivates the absence it was meant to overcome. What appears as fulfillment therefore renews the search. The attempt to satisfy desire becomes the mechanism through which its movement is perpetuated.

In this sense, the tragedy of desire can be understood as a doubling of the classical tragic structure. In line with Wilde and Shaw, both possibilities lead to the same impasse: not obtaining the desired object sustains longing, yet obtaining it reveals that the object cannot occupy the place assigned to it in fantasy. Desire is thus caught between two forms of failure, neither of which resolves the underlying lack. Both failure and fulfillment reproduce the same absence that sets desire in motion. Fairy tales may end with "And they lived happily ever after," but how such happiness could resolve desire remains unexplained.

Contemporary technological environments are particularly effective at concealing this doubled tragedy. Platforms such as Tinder sustain the movement of desire by continuously displacing it from one possible object to the next. Through this metonymic progression, both disappointment and apparent fulfillment are absorbed into the same ongoing search. A failed match leads to the next profile, while even a successful encounter rarely brings desire to rest, but instead redirects it toward the next potential partner.

This movement is closely tied to the opacity of desire itself. Because desire is mediated by the desire of the Other, it is never fully transparent to the subject. When a particular object fails, the subject cannot determine whether it was ever the right object, and therefore redirects the search. The movement from one object to the next reflects not only the impossibility of satisfaction but also the subject's uncertainty about what it wants.

In earlier social contexts, this uncertainty was often managed through external forms of mediation. Families or communities were assumed to know what constituted a suitable match. In some cases this took the form of arranged marriages governed by established norms and practices.

In modern societies, the responsibility for choosing a partner has increasingly shifted to the individual. Contemporary debates often frame this shift as a movement from social determination to individual autonomy. Yet from a Lacanian perspective, this opposition is misleading. Because desire is always mediated by the Other, the subject can never be certain that what it wants is fully its own. The question therefore remains unavoidable: How do we know what we really want?

Dating platforms such as Tinder appear to offer a technological response to this dilemma. They promise to support individual choice by matching users with partners who correspond to their preferences. In doing so, they resonate with ideas such as nudging and libertarian paternalism, where aspects of decision-making are delegated to systems that simplify selection.

Yet this apparent empowerment conceals a structural continuity. Where earlier the family or community functioned as matchmaker, this role is now increasingly taken over by algorithmic systems. The authority that orients desire shifts from social institutions to technological infrastructures. Here the Other no longer appears as a figure but as an environment.

What distinguishes contemporary algorithmic environments is therefore not the presence of mediation but the way in which it is reconfigurated and concealed. In this process, stable points of identification are loosened while their structuring role is obscured. Platforms such as Tinder increasingly occupy a position that structurally resembles the place of the Other: the site from which subjects receive indications about what is desirable and whom they should choose. Yet this authority does not appear as an external command. It appears as the neutral operation of a technological system that merely presents options and recommendations.

Precisely in this form lies its effectiveness. The environment quietly structures the horizon within which partners appear, while the subject experiences itself as freely navigating among them. The place of the Other has not disappeared; it has become infrastructural. Because this mediation is embedded in the technological environment itself, the question of who or what structures desire recedes from view. The subject continues to experience the choice as its own, even though the field in which desire moves is already algorithmically organized elsewhere. The structural split of the subject therefore remains, but technological mediation makes it easier to displace this condition.

Algorithmic environments do not resolve the tragedy of desire but reorganize the conditions under which it unfolds. They reshape how subjects position themselves in relation to others and to their own lack, and help explain why technological promises continue to resonate despite the impossibility of wholeness. By organizing encounters through profiles and algorithmic filtering, environments such as Tinder expose subjects to the gaze and desire of others and stage the question of what one wants and is wanted for.

These dynamics can be understood more precisely through Lacan's clinical structures. What is at stake is not a psychiatric diagnosis of users but the way different relations to lack are enacted and sustained within algorithmically mediated environments, and how these positions are intensified, displaced or reorganized through them.

Structural Relations to Lack in Technological Environments

The Psychotic Tech Mode: The Absorbed

In psychosis, the subject's relation to the Other is not symbolically mediated. As discussed earlier, this follows from the foreclosure of the Name-of-the-Father: the signifier that would normally anchor meaning and introduce separation does not take hold. As a result, the subject is neither properly inscribed in the symbolic order nor able to recognize the lack in the Other. It undergoes neither alienation nor separation and cannot establish a stable distance from the gaze, judgments and demands it encounters. What is missing is the mediation that would allow the subject to interpret and regulate this exposure. Rather than encountering the Other as Other and as lacking Other, the subject confronts it as immediate and overwhelming. The question of what the Other wants cannot be situated, and the subject is left without the symbolic coordinates that would stabilize its relation to it.

Seen through this lens, patterns in digital environments become more intelligible. Platforms organized around visibility and continuous feedback expose users to a field of evaluation in which appearance becomes central to recognition. Images, profiles and metrics intensify awareness of being seen and judged (Hanna et al. 2017; Trekels et al. 2018; Ward et al. 2016; Baker et al. 2019; Saiphoo and Vahedi 2019). Users often attempt to conform to perceived ideals and experience dissatisfaction when they fail to do so (Baker et al. 2019, 280; Bell et al. 2016; Brown and Tiggemann 2016; Fox and Rooney 2015).

In algorithmic environments, the psychotic structure takes shape as a position in which subjects are continuously exposed to evaluation without the symbolic resources needed to interpret or regulate it. To avoid clinical connotations, and to mark that this is not a pathology but a position generated and stabilized by environments that immerse subjects in an unmediated and opaque field of evaluation, eroding the distance needed to situate the Other and their own place in relation to it, I will refer to this position as *the absorbed*.

This continuous exposure to evaluation and the resulting sensitivity to being seen and judged are commonly framed in terms of self-esteem or social comparison. The psychotic position, here recast as the absorbed, does not replace these accounts but reframes them structurally. What appears as insecurity or comparison anxiety reflects a difficulty in establishing distance from the gaze of the Other. The absorbed is exposed to judgments it cannot fully interpret or stabilize and remains dependent on a field of evaluation that lacks clear symbolic mediation.

Environments such as Tinder intensify this condition. By organizing encounters through rapid sequences of profiles and simple gestures of approval or rejection, the platform amplifies exposure to the gaze of others while providing limited resources to interpret it. The abundance of potential partners and the constant feedback of matches or their absence heighten sensitivity to perceived judgment (Strübel and Petrie 2017; Heino et al. 2010, 434–438).

Viewed through the psychotic lens, the crucial issue is not merely comparison or objectification but the absorbed's increasing exposure to the gaze of the Other without symbolic mediation. It becomes increasingly dependent on external evaluations it cannot symbolically process or stabilize. When symbolic structures fail to provide distance from this gaze, the absorbed may become caught in an oscillation between identification with its online appearance and anxiety about how that appearance is judged.

This vulnerability can be further specified through Lacan's two substructures of psychosis: schizophrenia and paranoia. In schizophrenia, the absence of a symbolic boundary between self and Other makes it difficult to regulate or filter what comes from outside. Judgments and perceptions cannot be stabilized and may become overwhelming. In environments such as Tinder, where users are continuously exposed to profiles, evaluations and potential rejection, this may appear as a sense of being flooded by judgments that cannot be processed. Strübel (2023) notes that even users with initially high self-esteem may experience a diminished sense of self after repeated use (Strübel 2023, 11). The absorbed is thus left at the mercy of an opaque and fluctuating field of evaluation.

Another psychotic substructure is paranoia. Here the absence of symbolic mediation produces a distinct dynamic. Rather than being engulfed by the Other, the absorbed encounters it as a rival or threatening presence. Without a symbolic order to mediate social relations, interaction may become locked in dyadic confrontations marked by rivalry and suspicion. This again reflects the failure to inscribe the father's No, which would otherwise introduce a symbolic third and situate the absorbed within shared limits. Without such mediation, the absorbed struggles to move beyond direct confrontation. In the Tinder environment, where users constantly compare themselves and compete for attention, these dynamics may become especially pronounced. In more extreme cases, the absorbed may become fixed in a relation of persistent rivalry with an imagined Other experienced as inherently hostile and threatening.

The validation market on Tinder intensifies this dynamic, fostering a continuous cycle of judgment and comparison. The absorbed is exposed to a field of evaluations that it cannot regulate or interpret. Many report needing to take "breaks" from the app because it makes them feel bad (Strübel 2023, 11). This indicates how difficult it is to maintain a critical or reflective stance within the platform; distance seems possible only once one steps outside it. As one user puts it:

> I feel like I've started looking at people as disposable, as far as a partner goes. Scared to connect because there could be someone else out there who's better and I could be wasting my time with the wrong person. What's funny is everyone seems like the wrong person. Helped me realize my fear of commitment, or just my fear of attempting a relationship currently.
>
> (Man, 21 years old; in Strübel 2023, 11)

Seen through the psychotic lens, these experiences point to a broader structural dynamic. Tinder continuously exposes users to the gaze and judgment of others while offering few symbolic resources to interpret or stabilize them. What appears as a platform for facilitating encounters may therefore also function as an environment in which the absorbed is systematically exposed to the unmediated presence of the Other. In this respect, Tinder exemplifies a broader tendency of contemporary algorithmic environments, in which subjects confront fields of evaluation that operate without clear symbolic mediation.

The Perverse Tech Mode: The Pleaser

Disavowal characterizes the perverse structure. Unlike psychosis, the subject is inscribed into the symbolic order, yet it does not recognize that the Other itself is lacking. It sustains the Other as complete. In Lacanian terms, the subject undergoes alienation but not separation. Confronted with the loss of jouissance, it refuses to accept this loss and to translate it into desire. The result is a structural impasse: jouissance cannot be maintained, yet the loss required for desire is denied. The perverse response to this impasse is to position oneself as the object through which the Other's jouissance is realized. Rather than relating to an enigmatic and lacking Other, the subject assumes it knows what the Other wants and makes itself the object that satisfies it. In doing so, it secures a determinate place for itself and avoids the uncertainty that sustains desire.

Regardless of a person's motivation for using Tinder, the platform's strong emphasis on appearance makes users hypersensitive to how they appear to others. Strübel and Petrie (2017, 37) show that appearance-focused social media teach both male and female Tinder users to equate self-worth with sexualized appearance. These platforms encourage self-objectification to attract matches and promote the posting of sexualized images to seek validation (Meier and Gray 2014). The platform thus nudges the subject to experience itself and its body as objects meant to satisfy others.

Seen through the perverse lens, this dynamic reveals more than objectification alone. It shows how subjects are invited to occupy the position of the object through which the Other's enjoyment is realized. In algorithmic environments such as Tinder, this position is organized through technological infrastructures that simulate the gaze of an anonymous Other. What emerges is the difficulty of taking up a symbolic position, translating the value of the subject into something other than an extension for the Other, such as someone to be respected or admired.

In algorithmic environments, the perverse structure takes shape as a position in which subjects organize themselves as objects in response to signals of what is desired, without fully recognizing the lack that structures the Other. Following the earlier shift in terminology, I will refer to this position as *the pleaser*. This term captures how subjects align themselves with perceived demand and take up the role of the object meant to satisfy it.

Tinder's nudging mechanisms reinforce these dynamics. By organizing encounters around profiles, visual evaluation and the rapid gesture of swiping left or right, the platform continually invites users to present themselves as objects for the gaze of others. The pleaser is thus positioned within a technologically organized symbolic field of recognition, yet interaction remains confined to cycles of evaluation and validation. Rather than sustaining the uncertainty of the Other's desire, the pleaser attempts to satisfy it by presenting itself as the object the Other might want. In this way the pleaser remains alienated without achieving separation. Jouissance is sustained through validation rather than translated into desire. This fundamental trait runs through Lacan's subtypes of perversion: fetishism, masochism and sadism.

In fetishism, the subject is reduced, or reduces itself, to a thing that facilitates the jouissance of others. Rather than occupying a symbolic position in the desire of the Other, the subject becomes an object meant to satisfy it. Women in particular often report experiences that resonate with this dynamic when using Tinder:

> [I feel] very sad, guys treat me like meat, or an object (Woman, 19 years old).
>
> It made me feel horrible and disgusting. Like the only thing I am good for is my physical appearance, which I am not even that confident in. I felt like I was not worthy in any man's eyes as an intellectual, but solely there for his desires and pleasures (Woman, 24 years old). I feel that I am sometimes more self conscious of how I look because I know hundreds of men are constantly on there judging me by my appearance.
>
> (Woman, 24 years old) (in Strübel 2023, 10)

Such experiences of objectification are associated with lower self-esteem, higher psychological distress, anxiety, depression and a decline in overall self-perception and mental health (Hawes et al. 2020; Holtzhausen et al. 2020; Hanna et al. 2017).

Yet the perverse strategy of completing the Other inevitably fails. No object, however devotedly offered, can fill the lack that structures desire. This impossibility generates anxiety and pushes the subject to develop new ways of stabilizing the relation to the Other.

This dynamic becomes particularly visible in masochism and sadism. In masochism, the subject consciously "does anything for the sake of the jouissance of the Other" (Van Haute 2001, 243) while at an unconscious level aiming to push this enjoyment to the point where it becomes intolerable, thereby provoking the emergence of a law that would impose limits on it (Van Haute 2001, 244).

Tinder users often place themselves in environments structured by constant evaluation, where their worth becomes tied to how attractive they appear to others. Yet when users protest against being treated as mere "meat," they simultaneously signal a demand for symbolic recognition: to be acknowledged as more than an object, as a professional, an intellectual or a person with a life beyond appearance.

Sadism expresses the opposite configuration. Consciously, the sadist reduces "the victim to a mere means to the end of his or her own jouissance" (Van Haute 2001, 241). Unconsciously, however, the sadist likewise seeks the emergence of a law that would regulate this excessive enjoyment. Applied to Tinder, users who treat others as objects to consume may come to experience themselves as vehicles of the Other's desire, implicitly calling for limits to this dynamic. Several participants report needing to take breaks from Tinder because the experience leaves them feeling bad about themselves. As one user notes, "It is great for increasing validation through women, but can be unhealthy for self worth at times because it becomes almost addicting" (Man, 27 years old; in Strübel 2023, 11).

Across these variations, the central issue remains the same: finding a position for the subject that allows it to be something more than an imaginary object for the Other. Tinder's emphasis on appearance and rapid evaluation makes this dynamic particularly visible. Its algorithms continuously invite users to judge, measure and swipe left or right on one another. Similar dynamics increasingly characterize contemporary algorithmic environments more broadly. Systems that rank, filter and recommend subjects on the basis of data-driven metrics position individuals within fields of evaluation in which they are invited to present themselves as objects of attraction, performance or consumption. In this respect, algorithmic environments increasingly organize interaction in ways that resonate with the perverse structure, encouraging subjects to present themselves as objects capable of satisfying the desire of an anonymous Other. Within such environments, the pleaser is continuously reproduced as a position organized around anticipating and aligning with this demand. At the same time, the pleaser attempts to resist this reduction by presenting itself as more than a body, invoking professions, identities or personal narratives.

The Neurotic Tech Mode: The Seeker

Neurosis designates a position in which the subject is both constituted by the Other and confronted with its lack. Unlike psychosis, where neither alienation nor separation takes place, and perversion, where alienation is not followed by separation, neurosis involves both. The subject is inscribed into the symbolic order and recognizes the Law, yet also encounters the Other as lacking. The neurotic's mode of denial is repression. It accepts symbolic castration but pushes its implications into the unconscious, producing a split between conscious and unconscious, ego and subject. The impossibility of full jouissance is thus both acknowledged and disavowed. As Fink notes, the neurotic separates from the Other but does not succeed in "traversing the fantasy" (Fink 1997, 195). Fantasy veils the loss introduced by castration and sustains the belief that what was lost might still be recovered. The question "Che vuoi?" persists, but no answer holds: each apparent resolution gives way to renewed doubt. Neurosis is thus structured by an ongoing oscillation between expectation and dissatisfaction.

Seen through this lens, the dynamics of Tinder become particularly intelligible while also illustrating a broader pattern characteristic of algorithmic environments. The platform confronts users with the possibility that somewhere among an endless stream of profiles there might be the person who could resolve the question of desire. At the same time, the abundance of alternatives continually undermines this possibility. Each match appears provisional, each decision reversible. Users oscillate between attraction and hesitation, engagement and withdrawal. Empirical studies report uncertainty, fear of missing out and difficulty committing, precisely because new options are always available (Strübel 2023). What appears as indecision can thus be understood as the neurotic structure of desire: the persistent search for an object that might answer what one wants, combined with the impossibility of securing that answer.

In algorithmic environments, the neurotic structure takes shape as a position in which subjects remain caught in an ongoing circulation of options, sustained by the expectation that an object might yet resolve the question of desire. Following the earlier shift in terminology, I will refer to this position as *the seeker*. This term captures how subjects continue to search, compare and anticipate without arriving at a position that would stabilize desire.

Lacan distinguishes two principal substructures of neurosis: obsession and hysteria. In obsessional neurosis, the subject accepts the loss of jouissance yet continues to search for an object that might restore completeness. On Tinder, this appears as an endless search for the "right" match, accompanied by the suspicion that no match will suffice:

> I feel like I've started looking at people as disposable, as far as a partner goes. Scared to connect because there could be someone else out there who's better and I could be wasting my time with the wrong person. What's funny is everyone seems like the wrong person. Helped me realize my fear of commitment, or just my fear of attempting a relationship currently.
>
> (Man, 21 years old; in Strübel 2023, 11)

Here, potential partners are treated as candidates for the lost *object a*, yet each fails in advance. Because doubt cannot be resolved, the seeker continues to search even as it produces frustration or exhaustion.

The other main neurotic substructure, hysteria, is organized differently. Rather than seeking a definitive object, the hysteric sustains the question of the Other's desire. It continually asks what the Other wants and attempts to position itself in relation to that question without resolving it. This dynamic is echoed in many Tinder experiences:

> It is great for increasing validation through women, but can be unhealthy for self-worth at times because it becomes almost addicting.
>
> (Man, 27 years old; in Strübel 2023, 11)

> I use it to see how attractive people find me, and when I get a lot of matches I feel confident. If I don't then I will change my profile to see what will get me more matches.
>
> (Woman, 21 years old; in Strübel 2023, 11)

> I feel a bit more confident than I did before. I feel like I may have felt some validation from having the majority of people swipe right for my profile.
>
> (Woman, 27 years old; in Strübel 2023, 14)

The hysteric desires through the desire of the Other and repeatedly attempts to become the object that might answer it while keeping the question open. Unlike the pervert, who assumes certainty, the hysteric sustains uncertainty as such. The seeker thus remains oriented toward an answer that is never secured, sustaining the movement of desire itself.

Across these variations, the neurotic position is marked by a tension that cannot be resolved. The subject seeks recognition yet resists full absorption by the Other. Full validation would threaten the distance that sustains desire, while its absence reactivates the search. This tension could explain why some Tinder users, on the one hand, strive to appear as attractive and desirable as possible and, on the other, revolt when they feel reduced to mere "meat." The longing for wholeness is thus accompanied by equally strong strategies that prevent full absorption by the Other, whether through the obsessive postponement of commitment or through the hysteric's continual reopening of the question of the Other's desire.

This balance remains fragile. When oscillation intensifies, doubt may turn into despair. As one user expresses: "date 9, The last one has definitely opened a Pandora's box of emotions for me, forcing me to re-evaluate what the hell I want from Tinder and life" (Quora Accessed February 25, 2026).

With the sheer number of options, the ease of moving on, and the persistent sense that someone better might always be available, Tinder not only mirrors but intensifies this structure. Its algorithm continuously reorganizes the field of encounters, reopening the question of what one wants and who might provide the missing object. In this respect, Tinder exemplifies a broader tendency of algorithmic environments: by generating endless alternatives and comparisons, they keep the question of desire permanently unsettled. Within such environments, the seeker is continuously reproduced as a position sustained by comparison, anticipation and the deferral of resolution, sustaining doubt and, at times, pushing it toward despair.

Beyond Neurosis: The Question of Singularity in Algorithmic Systems

Psychosis, perversion and neurosis do not exhaust the field of relating to lack and castration. As Chapter 3 has shown, Lacan's later work opens the possibility of a position beyond neurosis. This position does not designate a cured subject. The question "Che vuoi?" and the struggles it entails do not disappear, nor is the relation to the Other overcome. What changes is its function. The subject no longer approaches the Other as the locus of a definitive answer but recognizes its own implication in the question that structures its desire. The question of desire is no longer treated as something that can be resolved, even after extensive searching, but as something to be sustained without closure. In neurosis, *object a* remains bound to the fantasy that an object might be found that would finally answer the subject's question; beyond neurosis, *object a* no longer appears as something that could complete the subject but as the structural remainder around which desire and enjoyment continue to circulate. It no longer promises wholeness but marks the gap that makes such wholeness impossible.

Singularity should therefore not be confused with autonomy in the sense of self-mastery or independence. Nothing in this movement abolishes division or eliminates lack. It designates an increased capacity to assume and navigate the constitutive incompleteness of subjectivity (see also McGowan 2024).

Algorithmic systems can intensify the search for completion but also expose its impossibility. Against this background, the structural responses discussed are not psychological types but heuristic figures that clarify how subjects relate to lack within technological environments. They should be understood not as better or worse but as different ways of inhabiting lack that vary in stability and livability.

This distinction is visualized in Figure 5.1, which presents the four structural positions in relation to one another. As introduced in the preceding sections, I refer to these positions as the absorbed, the pleaser, the seeker and the singular. While the first three terms translate Lacan's clinical structures into the context of algorithmic environments, the singular is retained to designate the position beyond neurosis, which does not carry the same clinical connotation.

The aim here is to show how these positions relate to one another and how each organizes a distinct way of responding to lack within algorithmic environments. The absorbed corresponds to the psychotic position, where the subject lacks symbolic mediation and is exposed to the Real, becoming engulfed in algorithmic feedback, a configuration marked by low livability. The pleaser designates the perverse position, in which the subject organizes itself as the instrument of the Other's enjoyment, taking up the role of object while simultaneously attempting to evade it – a fragile and difficult position to sustain. The seeker captures the neurotic

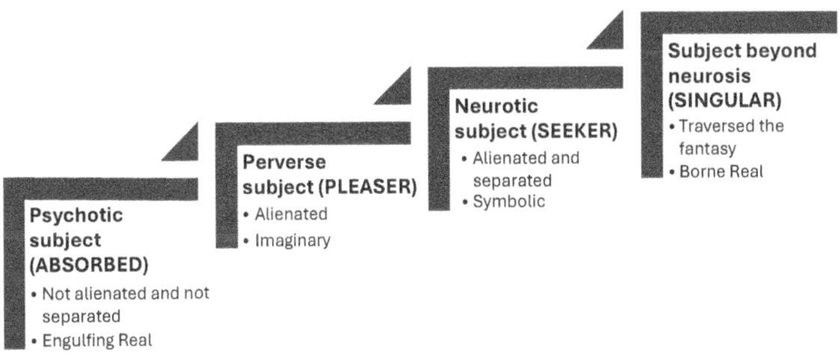

Figure 5.1 Four structural positions of the subject.

position: here the subject remains situated within the symbolic order yet is caught in a circulation of options, governed by the fantasy that an object might one day answer the question of the Other's desire, offering relative stability while remaining unsettled. The singular marks the position beyond neurosis, where the subject no longer seeks to overcome lack through the promise of completion but begins to bear the impossibility around which subjectivity itself is organized, designating a different mode of stability grounded in an ongoing, experimental engagement with lack.

Algorithmic environments such as Tinder may reinforce established ways of relating to lack, but they can also make their structure increasingly visible. They do not simply determine how subjects appear; they function as sites where subjects experiment with self-presentation, respond to algorithmic feedback and position themselves in relation to the gaze of the Other. In this sense, they do not necessarily reproduce the dynamics of psychosis, perversion and neurosis but may also open space for different modes of subjectivation. It is within this tension that the question of singularity acquires renewed relevance and will be taken up in the following chapter. The issue is therefore not how subjects might become whole through technological environments but whether these environments can become sites where subjects learn to inhabit their lack in their own way.

6 Designing for Singularity

Singularity arises not from overcoming lack but from taking ownership of the question of what one wants. This returns us to the central problem of this book: how contemporary technologies reorganize the subject's relation to desire and the promise of wholeness. In algorithmic environments that anticipate, track and modulate desire, platforms do not merely mediate subjectivity but shape how subjects relate to others and to the Other, and how what one wants takes form and persists. Designing for singularity therefore turns on how these environments structure the conditions under which subjects confront their lack and the impossibility of completion.

This chapter proceeds in four steps. It first analyzes how the shift from desire to drive takes shape within algorithmic environments that continuously solicit, capture and redirect the subject's investments. It then examines how responsive computational systems that seem to speak in the place of the Big Other return with renewed force, intensifying its authority while unsettling and potentially disrupting the fragile emergence of singularity. It next turns to experiments in algorithmic singularity, examining how these dynamics unfold in concrete technological settings, taking Tinder as a paradigmatic case. Finally, it turns to love in the context of algorithmic environments as a possible site for singularity.

From Desire to Drive

Desire, as structured lack, does not culminate in fulfillment but persists in its movement from object to object, sustained by the impossibility of completion. The drive marks a different relation to this lack: no longer oriented toward resolving it but sustained in a repetitive movement that no longer seeks an answer. The question, then, is how this shift becomes possible within technological environments. Do algorithmic systems merely intensify the promise of fulfillment, reinforcing the positions associated with the clinical structures, or do they also open a space in which

DOI: 10.4324/9781042010912-6

subjects can sustain their division differently, no longer seeking to overcome it but to relate to it otherwise?

Two responses can be set aside. One consists in seeking renewed orientation in an older symbolic order by withdrawing from algorithmic environments altogether. Digital detoxes, abandoning dating applications or nostalgic appeals to more stable forms of recognition belong to this category. Such gestures may offer temporary relief from continuous comparison and exposure, yet they leave the underlying economy of desire intact. The subject continues to seek reassurance in a symbolic order expected to provide stable coordinates of meaning, authority and recognition, even as these coordinates no longer fully hold.

A second possibility consists in remaining within algorithmic environments while reproducing the structural positions associated with psychosis, perversion and neurosis. Dating platforms and other visibility-driven environments intensify these dynamics by amplifying exposure, encouraging self-objectification for the Other's gaze and sustaining cycles of doubt, optimization and evaluation. Here the technological environment does not transform the relation to lack but accelerates familiar strategies of denial, disavowal and endless questioning.

What remains is a third possibility. Rather than withdrawing or becoming absorbed by logics of optimization and comparison, subjects may begin to experiment with inhabiting their mediated condition differently. This does not mean escaping mediation or recovering an authentic self prior to it. It involves recognizing that subjectivity is itself constituted through circuits of anticipation, misrecognition and repetition that algorithmic environments render difficult to ignore.

Under such conditions, encounters are no longer organized primarily around success or failure but begin to expose the persistence of the subject's own investments. Desire does not disappear, but its demand for resolution loses urgency as enjoyment becomes organized around the movement itself rather than the attainment of a definitive object.

In this sense, algorithmic environments can function as paradoxical laboratories of subjectivation. They intensify comparison, evaluation and uncertainty yet also render visible the repetitive structures through which the subject seeks recognition and completion. The acceleration of matches, recommendations and feedback loops makes perceptible what earlier symbolic contexts allowed to be deferred: the structural impossibility at the heart of desire. Singularity arises not from escaping these environments but from experimenting with how one's desire circulates within them.

These possibilities remain fragile. The same infrastructures that render repetition visible continuously reintroduce pressures of quantification, visibility and self-optimization. The loosening of fixed symbolic coordinates is accompanied by an intensified demand to position oneself within shifting regimes of evaluation. Singularity emerges, if at all, within this tension.

This ambivalence deepens as algorithmic systems begin not only to structure the field of desire but to approximate the position from which the subject is addressed. Increasingly, they do more than sort, recommend or predict. They simulate responsiveness, interpretation and recognition, appearing to occupy the place of the Other as locus of authority, knowledge and desire. The problem is therefore no longer only how subjects relate to their lack within these environments but what happens when the environments themselves seem to speak. It is this intensification of the Other that the next section examines.

When the Algorithmic Other Speaks

Contemporary data- and algorithm-driven environments do not merely reorganize the spaces in which desire circulates. They destabilize the symbolic frameworks that historically provided relatively stable coordinates for identity, authority and recognition. This destabilization does not simply result from the disappearance of norms or institutions. More fundamentally, algorithmic environments unsettle the experience that symbolic orientation rests on a stable Big Other. Through continuous processes of ranking, prediction, personalization and recalibration, they render visible that what counts as valuable, desirable or legitimate is not grounded in a fixed order but incessantly produced within shifting regimes of evaluation. What once appeared as a relatively consistent framework increasingly presents itself as provisional, revisable and technologically mediated.

For the subject, this transformation does not primarily produce emancipation but a more unsettling exposure. As the assumption erodes that there exists an authority who ultimately knows what one should be or desire, orientation itself becomes contingent. Desire is less securely mediated by symbolic reference points that once rendered lack intelligible and bearable. The subject can no longer defer the question of its position to an already given order but is increasingly compelled to confront the indeterminate character of its own desire without the reassurance that symbolic authority will stabilize it.

Yet this opening does not automatically lead to singular self-formation. The erosion of established coordinates can just as readily produce disorientation, anxiety and an intensified search for new loci of guidance. When traditional Big Others lose their authority, the desire for orientation does not disappear but can become more urgent.

Precisely within this space of weakened guarantees, technological environments generate a new intensification of the Other. Algorithmic systems no longer function merely as infrastructures that sort, recommend or predict. They increasingly simulate responsiveness, interpretation and forms of recognition. Interfaces that generate language, anticipate questions and produce seemingly meaningful replies can come to occupy a position structurally analogous to the locus traditionally attributed to the Big Other. Subjects may experience themselves as addressed by systems whose authority derives less from institutional legitimacy than from the impression that there exists a technological instance capable of knowing, responding and guiding.

The emergence of large language models such as ChatGPT exemplifies this transformation. These systems do not simply mediate communication; they begin to shape the conditions under which subjects articulate themselves. By offering fluent and context-sensitive responses, they can appear to preempt the uncertainty historically condensed in the question "Che vuoi?" Instead of encountering this question as a structurally unsettling confrontation, users may increasingly experience it as a practical problem that can be operationalized, optimized or technologically resolved.

This development is no longer confined to exceptional contexts. ChatGPT has rapidly become an ordinary companion in practices of writing, presenting and responding. Emails, formal documents, holiday cards, résumés, cover letters and social media interactions are increasingly shaped through algorithmically assisted language. What once required the subject to assume the risk of articulation is now frequently delegated to responsive computational systems. As these systems move from peripheral instruments to intimate companions in processes of self-presentation and recognition, they reinforce the impression that the question of one's desire need not be assumed but can be managed.

Yet this seemingly personalized assistance conceals a decisive paradox. On the one hand, algorithmic systems adapt to the user's tone and preferences, producing the experience of individualized support. On the other hand, their formulations are drawn from large-scale datasets that stabilize what is broadly recognizable as persuasive, appropriate or desirable communication. Personalization thus simultaneously functions as normalization. Through growing reliance on such systems, subjects risk aligning their own voice with collectively sedimented patterns. The distinction between singular articulation and data-shaped templates becomes blurred. The system no longer functions as a neutral instrument but participates in structuring how recognition is sought and granted. As this mediation intensifies, the space in which desire can be assumed as one's own begins to contract.

From a Lacanian perspective, this development does not reinforce a single clinical configuration but reconfigures the field of subjectivation. What begins as a supportive intensification of neurotic mediation may, under conditions of increasing reliance, shift toward perverse compliance and, in more extreme forms, toward a psychotic erosion of the distance that sustains subjectivity.

Initially, this often takes the form of a renewed neurotic orientation. The subject continues to doubt, hesitate and compare its own formulations with those generated by the machine. Yet this seeking increasingly unfolds within coordinates already anticipated by algorithmic systems. The question does not disappear but becomes dependent on an authority that appears consistently competent and contextually attuned. Doubt is not abolished but reorganized into a recursive circuit in which the subject repeatedly turns to the technological Other to stabilize its position, calibrate what it should say and anticipate what might be desired. Doubt risks losing its disruptive force and becoming a managed moment within an ongoing process of optimization, a dynamic that leaves no escape from the position of the *seeker*.

Within this dynamic, perverse tendencies can emerge. As hesitation becomes integrated into algorithmic circuits of consultation, subjects may begin not only to rely on systems such as ChatGPT but to orient themselves toward satisfying the standards these systems appear to embody. Users increasingly emulate its fluent and polished style. The questioning position can shift toward a pleasing position in which the subject anticipates and performs what is presumed desirable. Expression becomes less a struggle with the opacity of desire and more a performance aligned with expected norms. The subject risks becoming captured in the position of the *pleaser*, organizing itself as the object best suited to secure recognition within regimes that reward coherence, fluency and adaptability.

The psychotic danger emerges when even this minimal distance between subject and technological locus of address begins to dissolve. When systems appear capable of scripting responses, anticipating preferences or articulating desires on behalf of the user, the processes of alienation and separation through which subjectivity ordinarily takes shape can erode. What begins as mediation can become substitution. The question of desire is no longer encountered as open but as already answered. As algorithmically generated formulations appear more coherent or authoritative than one's own divided articulations, the subject may begin to trust these outputs more than its own uncertainty. Dependence approaches fusion. In this limit, the subject risks sliding into the position of the *absorbed*, a movement from which it can no longer extricate itself, as symbolic mediation collapses and one's own desire becomes indistinguishable from the discourse that speaks through it.

This movement becomes most radical when algorithmic communication loops begin to operate with decreasing reference to a speaking subject. Messages generated with technological assistance are read, interpreted, reformulated and answered through comparable systems, producing circuits in which discourse circulates in a quasi-autonomous manner. What is at stake is no longer alignment with machinic fluency but a reconfiguration of the symbolic function of address itself. Communication risks becoming self-sustaining, less dependent on a divided subject who assumes a position in speech. The Other no longer appears as a locus structured by distance and lack but as an absorptive field of algorithmic articulation that seems capable of speaking without the subject.

Yet precisely where this apparent closure becomes most radical, another possibility emerges. The very systems that seem to render the subject superfluous can expose their own inconsistency. Moments of opacity, misalignment or so-called hallucination interrupt the illusion that the technological Other truly knows. When algorithmic discourse reveals its contingent and self-generating character, the subject is again confronted with the impossibility of delegating the question of desire. What appeared as a seamless substitute turns into a renewed encounter with uncertainty.

In such moments, guidance gives way to disturbance. The promise of certainty folds back upon itself. The attempt to eliminate uncertainty by outsourcing desire confronts the subject with the fact that this question cannot be delegated. What returns is not the stability of a former symbolic order but the irreducible openness of one's own position.

The intensification of the algorithmic Other does not foreclose singular self-formation but radicalizes its stakes. The subject is drawn deeper into circuits of technological anticipation, only to encounter the limits of what such anticipation can deliver. The more convincingly the machine appears to know, the more disruptive the moment in which this knowledge falters. It is within this oscillation between seductive certainty and structural impossibility that a new terrain of subjectivation takes shape.

What emerges is a more demanding task: remaining within technologically intensified fields of address without allowing them to close the question of desire. The subject must inhabit an environment that anticipates its speech, while recognizing that no machinic articulation can assume its position.

It is within this tension, between the promise that desire can be calculated and the recurring experience that it cannot, that the possibility of more *singular* forms of engagement appears. The next section turns to this fragile opening.

Experiments in Algorithmic Singularity

After Symbolic Stability

After symbolic stability has eroded, subjectivity does not find itself in a space of pure openness. Traditional frameworks that once offered relatively durable coordinates for identity and desire are indeed weakened, yet this erosion does not leave subjects in a silent void. On the contrary, they find themselves immersed in an incessant circulation of responses, recommendations and evaluations: buy this, choose that, improve yourself in this way. Algorithmic environments do not simply withdraw the coordinates through which desire was once mediated. They multiply them. Rankings, recommendations, predictions and suggestions incessantly offer provisional answers to questions that were previously sustained by relatively durable symbolic frameworks. The subject is therefore not left without guidance but confronted with an excess of it.

Nowhere is this more palpable than in algorithmically generated partner suggestions, which carry the intensified promise that even desire itself can be anticipated, optimized and successfully guided. Thus, even as symbolic guarantees become unstable, technologically mediated systems continue to offer seemingly persuasive answers to the question of what one should say, want or become. In this altered constellation, orientation no longer derives from a stable order presumed to know but from a dispersed and technologically mediated circulation of responses that both attract and unsettle. Subjectivity begins to take shape within a landscape in which symbolic reference points are weakened, while the pressure to position oneself intensifies.

This constellation produces a profoundly ambivalent condition for subjectivation. The weakening of stable authorities and symbolic guarantees does not suspend the demand to take a position but radicalizes it. The subject is increasingly compelled to respond, to choose and to articulate itself even when the coordinates that might justify and sustain such articulation remain uncertain. Algorithmic environments and AI systems therefore do not simply disorient. They generate a condition in which orientation must be produced continuously rather than presupposed. Desire is no longer negotiated within relatively enduring symbolic frameworks but is repeatedly brought into play through situational prompts, provisional cues and technologically mediated invitations to act.

This multiplication of technologically mediated responses is further intensified by the emergence of generative AI systems capable of producing linguistically articulated suggestions, interpretations, and affective cues in real time. Large language models do not merely extend existing recommendation logics but contribute to the experience of inhabiting an increasingly articulate technological field that appears to anticipate possible formulations of desire in advance. The erosion of symbolic stability is thus accompanied not by silence but by an environment that speaks more insistently and seemingly personally than ever.

This transformation also alters the temporal structure of subjectivation. Instead of unfolding within horizons shaped by tradition, prohibition and deferred recognition, the subject encounters a mode of temporality marked by perpetual updating and anticipatory recalibration. Responses are expected in real time and immediately folded back into new cycles of suggestion and evaluation. Increasingly, these cycles are shaped not only by recommendation systems and ranking mechanisms but also by generative interfaces that actively participate in the articulation of profiles, preferences and conversational styles. Desire risks becoming entrained to these feedback rhythms, leaving diminished space for the slower work of assuming lack. Symbolic authority is therefore not simply weakened but redistributed across a dispersed technological field, intensified by systems that appear to "speak" in increasingly personalized and anticipatory ways, keeping the subject in motion while withholding any final point of orientation.

Under these conditions, faster cycles of response and recalibration do not lead subjects to step back from algorithmic environments. They tend instead to intensify involvement in the very circuits that promise orientation. Many remain caught in recurrent patterns of comparison, anticipation, optimization and renewed adjustment, continuing to seek guidance through recommendation systems, visibility metrics and generative prompts that seem to prefigure what they might say or want. Under such conditions, the destabilization of symbolic order can give rise not to emancipation but to subtle processes of degeneration, in which searching hardens into adaptation or erodes the distance through which desire can be assumed.

Only intermittently do more reflexive modes of engagement emerge. In such moments, subjects begin to experiment with inhabiting mediation rather than simply oscillating within its demands. These practices do not constitute an exit from technologically organized regimes of recognition. They signal fragile shifts in which subjects start to recognize that their own self-relation is shaped through, rather than merely constrained by, these environments.

This development echoes a Hegelian logic of recognition. For Hegel, self-consciousness emerges not by escaping the relations that shape it but by coming to recognize itself within them (Hegel 2018, §§178–184). What initially appears as an external determination gradually becomes intelligible as a constitutive condition of one's own formation.

In algorithmic environments, a similar movement can be discerned. Subjects gradually come to recognize that the technological frameworks through which they seek orientation do not merely constrain them from the outside but participate in shaping how they come to understand themselves and what they take themselves to desire. Singular subjectivation therefore cannot consist in a nostalgic attempt to recover an imagined position outside mediation. It requires an active assumption of one's technologically conditioned situation and a growing awareness that the articulation of desire always takes place within mediated fields of recognition.

The increasing integration of generative systems sharpens this dynamic in a specific way. By reducing the experiential distance between subject and algorithmic environment, such systems can create the impression that mediation is being overcome, as if desire could now be directly articulated with technological assistance. Yet precisely this proximity renders mediation more visible. When generative interfaces propose formulations, shape self-presentations or anticipate possible responses, they expose how the subject's voice is already formed within symbolic and technical structures. Rather than resolving uncertainty, these systems can intensify the experience that desire does not originate from a self-grounded interiority but is continuously shaped through relations, infrastructures and interpretive frameworks.

This becomes particularly evident in everyday user practices. Empirical research shows that users frequently modify profiles, rewrite descriptions and curate images in response to visibility metrics and algorithmic recommendations (Fox and Rooney 2015; Ward et al., 2016; Strübel 2023). These adjustments might suggest an increasing awareness of mediation. Yet in most instances they remain embedded in a predominantly neurotic economy of recognition. They are driven less by reflexive experimentation than by the hope that more precise self-presentation, improved timing or increasingly strategic interaction will stabilize one's desirability. Rather than assuming lack, optimization keeps alive the fantasy of its resolution.

Only in a smaller range of more reflexive engagements does this logic begin to shift. Here, subjects no longer approach algorithmic infrastructures primarily as authorities presumed to know but begin to treat them as environments whose logics can be inhabited, displaced and partially reworked. What changes is not the presence of mediation but the relation to it.

Certain strands of feminist, queer and critical digital practices make this shift particularly visible (Hobbs, Owen and Gerber 2017). By unsettling norms from within the infrastructures that sustain them, they expose the contingency of regimes of desirability. In doing so, they open spaces in which these norms can be negotiated rather than simply followed. Yet such disruptions remain fragile. Singular gestures are quickly ranked, categorized and normalized, reabsorbed into the very circuits they momentarily interrupt.

What becomes visible in these dynamics is the structural ambivalence of algorithmic mediation itself. The same infrastructures that render the contingency of desire perceptible simultaneously channel this insight back into new regimes of visibility, comparison and evaluation. Reflexive distance does not simply escape these circuits but is itself drawn into them. The possibility of a different relation to desire therefore arises not outside algorithmic environments but within their tensions.

For this reason, the emancipatory promise of experimentation remains structurally precarious. Attempts to escape dominant symbolic orders may inadvertently install new authorities. After symbolic stability, subjectivation unfolds in a field where orientation is incessantly produced yet never fully reliable.

Singularity therefore acquires a more exacting meaning. It can no longer rely on the fantasy of stepping outside regimes of recognition. Rather, it concerns the capacity to sustain separation within mediation itself.

Traversing the Fantasy

Algorithmic environments do not abolish lack; rather, they tend to redistribute its experiential pressure by supplying increasingly plausible articulations of who one might be and what one might want. Rankings, recommendations and predictive suggestions sustain the impression that orientation can always be refined further. At the same time, the economic and operational logics of these environments rarely aim at resolving longing itself. Their functioning depends on the continued circulation of desire. What they offer are therefore not answers that bring desire to rest but sequences of provisional formulations that keep the subject engaged and affectively invested in ongoing interaction. The massive investments in attention engineering and behavioral optimization testify to this structural interest in prolonging participation within algorithmic circuits rather than concluding them.

The growing integration of large language models and generative systems further intensifies this dual constellation. By suggesting descriptions, anticipating preferences, modeling conversational tone and simulating possible relational trajectories, such systems increasingly give the impression that algorithmic mediation can deliver ever more precise and definitive answers to what one wants and who one might become. They do not merely filter or rank existing options but actively participate in shaping how intentions are formulated, how compatibility is imagined and how encounters are evaluated in real time. In this way the technological field appears to reduce uncertainty step by step, offering increasingly convincing approximations of fulfillment. Yet this very refinement also deepens and prolongs the user's investment. Each seemingly more accurate articulation generates further prompts for adjustment, continuation and renewed engagement. The environment thus appears to know desire in advance while simultaneously ensuring that its resolution remains just out of reach. What is multiplied are ever more persuasive formulations of completion, not completion itself. The promise of definitive answers is technologically intensified at the very moment it is structurally deferred. This promise of fulfillment and its structural nonrealization is therefore not a weakness of AI but a central condition of its success.

This dual movement finds its echo within the subject and the very structure of its desire. On the one hand, subjects remain driven to seek orientation and recognition, repeatedly engaging with promises of answers that might stabilize their longing. On the other hand, they never fully reach, nor entirely wish to reach, the point of definitive fulfillment. The unconscious sabotage of realized desire can be understood as a defense against the loss of subjective division itself. Complete satisfaction would suspend the very movement that sustains subjectivity. To encounter a fully satisfying answer would risk confronting the implication that desire, once fulfilled, would coincide with its own disappearance. The search therefore persists in a paradoxical form, sustained both by the attraction of potential resolution and by the structural necessity for such resolution to remain out of reach. It is precisely within this tension between algorithmic guidance and existential uncertainty, between the promise of orientation and the persistence of lack, that this paradox takes shape.

Under post-symbolic conditions, subjects may position themselves differently within this fragile constellation. Some remain absorbed in cycles of optimization and reassurance. Others begin to recognize how algorithmic environments shape their expectations, subtly nudge their orientations and frame the very terms through which they experience themselves as desiring beings. This recognition can disclose not only the workings of technological influence but also the structure of one's own longing.

Such insight may mark the beginning of a shift that can be described, in Lacanian terms, as a movement from desire toward drive. The subject does not abandon the search for connection, nor does longing disappear. What changes is the way its movement is inhabited. Engagement is no longer organized by the neurotic expectation that fulfillment will stabilize identity, but rather by an increased capacity to remain involved in circuits of attraction, tension, repetition and encounter without requiring that they culminate in resolution.

Within this altered orientation, *object a* comes into view not as a goal to be attained but as a cause that sustains investment precisely through its elusiveness. Desire continues to circulate, yet its repetitive movement is no longer experienced solely as frustration. It may also become the site of a certain satisfaction in circling around what cannot be integrated into a stable image of completion. The shift toward drive thus entails the capacity to remain within the impossibility of definitive fulfillment without converting this impossibility into resignation. As Fink has suggested, enjoyment may emerge not from closure but from sustaining the circuit itself.

The proliferation of generative mediation can paradoxically facilitate such repositioning. As algorithmic suggestions increasingly intervene in self-presentation and relational exchange, they render more perceptible the fact that subjectivity is formed within mediated environments and that an unmediated relation to oneself or to others is structurally impossible. What first appears as external guidance may thus come to be recognized as a constitutive condition rather than an external constraint.

Under these conditions, the question is no longer how to escape mediation but how to remain within the circuits that organize desire without demanding that they resolve it. Technological environments appear as intrinsically ambivalent: they enable processes of self-formation while simultaneously narrowing the space in which singular positions can be enacted. Recognizing this ambivalence does not resolve the tension, but it can shift the subject's relation to it. Algorithmic systems begin to appear less as authorities that must be satisfied and more as dynamics that can be observed, negotiated and at times strategically appropriated.

In this light, singular self-formation arises not from withdrawing from algorithmic mediation but from remaining within its circuits without treating them as promises of wholeness. The subject comes to recognize that longing persists because fulfillment cannot be secured, and that this persistence itself constitutes the movement through which subjectivity is enacted. To take up desire through drive therefore means continuing the search while relinquishing the demand that it must finally come to an end, allowing a distinct form of enjoyment to emerge in the persistence of longing itself rather than in the lost promise of full jouissance.

Singular self-formation therefore requires a repositioning on the side of the subject. Algorithmic environments continually invite users to approach mediated encounters as steps toward eventual completion. A more singular positioning becomes possible when these environments are instead approached as constitutive elements of the relational field rather than as hidden guarantors of fulfillment. Orientation, experimentation and engagement can then take place without the expectation that any configuration of mediation will resolve the structural tension of desire. What changes is not participation in technologically organized contexts but the subjective mode in which their operations are inhabited. Algorithmic mediation increasingly appears less as a source of definitive answers and solutions and more as a terrain within which subjects can explore how desire persists in the absence of guarantees.

Alongside this subjective repositioning, a further question emerges concerning the environments themselves. If singularity involves learning to inhabit mediated conditions without converting them into promises of wholeness, it becomes pertinent to ask whether algorithmic infrastructures can be configured in ways that make such repositioning more thinkable and more feasible. Rather than primarily intensifying cycles of optimization, prediction and behavioral steering, technological design might also open spaces for reflexive distance, temporal slowing or encounters that foreground contingency rather than conceal it. The issue at stake is therefore not only how subjects relate to mediation but how mediation might be shaped to support singular modes of self-formation.

The following section will illustrate this interplay between the subject's repositioning and the redesign of algorithmic environments by turning to the paradigmatic case of Tinder. Precisely because the choice of a partner carries such existential weight, users often become especially receptive to algorithmic guidance, investing trust in its capacity to orient desire and reduce uncertainty. This heightened sensitivity makes visible how fragile and demanding it is to navigate between reliance on technological mediation and the assumption of one's own lack, thereby offering a particularly clear site for examining how singular self-formation may either be constrained or enabled within algorithmically structured conditions of recognition.

A Lacanian Tinder

Attempts to design for singularity inevitably encounter a paradox. Precisely because technologically mediated environments increasingly organize the conditions under which desire unfolds, the question arises whether these environments might also be shaped in ways that allow subjects to relate differently to their lack. Were algorithmic systems to eliminate ambiguity altogether, they would not enable singular self-formation but foreclose it. Designing for singularity therefore requires cultivating forms of mediation that orient without stabilizing, guide without determining and structure encounters without resolving the lack that animates them.

Tinder condenses the contemporary tension between technologically mediated orientation and the structural instability of desire in a particularly acute form. The search for an intimate partner is not simply another domain of choice but one in which expectations of recognition, fulfillment and existential confirmation converge. Precisely because partner selection carries the promise of finally "getting the whole package," users become especially receptive to algorithmic guidance that appears to reduce uncertainty and increase the likelihood of eventual completion. In this sense, dating apps like Tinder function as laboratories in which the fragile negotiation between longing, projection and technological mediation becomes visible.

On Tinder, algorithmic matching does not resolve the divided structure of subjectivity but reorganizes how this division is experienced and negotiated. Curated profiles, compatibility scores and ranked suggestions frame existential lack as if it were a technical problem awaiting optimization. The platform thereby assumes the role of a contemporary Big Other that appears to know what one should desire and whom one should choose, gradually reshaping the positions from which users relate to themselves and to others. In engagement with this presumed authority, some subjects begin to align themselves closely with algorithmic cues, treating them not merely as suggestions but as increasingly credible indicators of what their desire ought to be. Others increasingly commodify their own presentation in order to remain visible within competitive regimes of desirability. Many remain caught in cycles of comparison, hesitation and renewed searching, hoping that more refined interaction strategies will eventually stabilize their position in relation to the desire of the Other.

These dynamics are further intensified as generative systems become integrated into everyday dating practices. Profiles are edited through large language models, conversational tones are modeled in advance, and relational trajectories are imaginatively rehearsed with technological assistance. In this way the platform begins to mediate not only encounters with potential partners but also the articulation of desire itself. The technological field increasingly appears capable of anticipating intention and smoothing out uncertainty, thereby strengthening the impression that existential ambiguity can be progressively reduced through better data, better matching or better communication.

At precisely this point, the question shifts from diagnosis to intervention. If singular self-formation requires subjects to assume their lack rather than displace it onto algorithmic guarantees, the issue becomes how the design of dating environments might support such repositioning. The question is not whether mediation can be eliminated but how its experiential logic can be transformed. Instead of reinforcing the fantasy that optimization will lead to completion, platforms such as Tinder could be configured to expose contingency, slow down circuits of consumption and sustain encounters that remain structurally unresolved.

A first design principle can be formulated as *resisting Tinder as Big Other*. Within Tinder's matching architecture, the algorithm often appears to "know" which profiles matter, which encounters are promising and which desires deserve to be pursued. Suggested matches, ranking sequences and patterns of visibility quietly shape the user's orientation, creating the impression that compatibility has already been assessed in advance. A Lacanian reconfiguration would aim to weaken this experiential authority. Tinder could stage moments in which the arbitrariness of recommendations becomes perceptible, interrupt the expectation that each profile represents progress toward fulfillment, or introduce encounters that fall outside established preference patterns. Such disruptions create symbolic distance between the user and the imagined knowledge of the system. Desire can then reappear not as something to be decoded through Tinder's suggestions but as a question that returns to the subject in the very act of swiping, pausing or choosing to engage.

Once this presumption of algorithmic knowledge is unsettled, a second design principle comes into view: *resisting Tinder as marketplace*. Tinder's swipe logic organizes partner seeking as a rapid sequence of visual comparisons in which attraction is constantly recalibrated across an apparently endless supply of profiles. Users are subtly encouraged to treat encounters as optimizable choices within a competitive field of desirability. A Lacanian redesign would seek to transform the lived rhythm of swiping itself. Profiles might unfold more gradually, interaction might be required before further evaluation becomes possible, or moments of enforced pause could disrupt the flow of consecutive selections. Such conditions slow the expectation of instant clarity and complicate the reduction of attraction to a stable preference. Instead of experiencing an abundance of interchangeable options, the user is confronted with the more demanding task of situating oneself in relation to another subject whose desire remains uncertain. Attraction begins to circulate less as rapid elimination and more as a temporally extended process structured by hesitation, curiosity and symbolic mediation.

From this altered rhythm of encounter, a third design principle becomes thinkable: *disrupting Tinder as a machine of wholeness*. Tinder culturally stages matching as if the right partner could finally bring existential lack to resolution. A Lacanian reconfiguration would instead sustain relational situations in which incompleteness remains visible and operative. Matches might develop through partial self-disclosure, shared activities within the application or exchanges that unfold across longer temporal arcs, preventing the too rapid fixing of what the other is taken to mean or represent. In such experiences the user gradually discovers that the aim is not to secure a perfectly compatible partner but to remain engaged in a relation that does not eliminate division. Desire then shifts its organization: rather than striving toward definitive fulfillment, it persists through renewed involvement in moments of attraction, hesitation and ambiguity, moving closer to the repetitive, circuitous satisfaction characteristic of drive.

From this perspective, the idea of a Lacanian Tinder application does not function as a concrete design blueprint but as a philosophical provocation that renders visible how technologically organized encounters might be reconfigured. The question is not how to implement a fixed set of features but how to transform the experiential logic of the platform itself. This would involve making algorithmic mediation more perceptible, interrupting the rapid circulation of profiles as consumable options and loosening the expectation of definitive compatibility. In this way, Tinder could shift from a space primarily oriented toward validation and optimization to one that sustains encounters with the persistence of lack. The aim is not to remove mediation but to make its limits visible so that users can no longer rely on the platform as if it knew their desire, but must assume their position within the encounters it organizes.

Yet the limits of design must remain clearly acknowledged. No arrangement of technological affordances can produce singularity as a guaranteed outcome or ensure more distinct forms of attachment. At most, a differently configured environment might create conditions in which reflexive confrontation with lack becomes more likely and in which the temporal openness necessary for desire to continue circulating is less easily foreclosed. Whether such conditions foster singular self-formation ultimately depends on how users take them up in practice, how they respond to moments of friction and how they engage the absence of definitive answers within digitally mediated encounters.

In this fragile negotiation between the promise of completion and the acceptance of irreducible incompleteness, the horizon of relating begins to shift. The search for a partner no longer revolves around finding someone who provides an answer, but becomes an encounter between two subjects who recognize that neither can complete the other. Where such encounters take the form of love – a notion taken up more explicitly in the following section – love no longer appears as the outcome of optimization but as a mode of relation that unfolds through contingency, misunderstanding and sustained engagement. It takes shape not through optimal alignment or shared compatibility but through the risky capacity to let desire persist where no algorithm can guarantee or complete it.

Love as Singularity

Having traced how algorithmic environments reshape desire, and how singularity emerges by inhabiting rather than overcoming lack, the question of love now comes into view. It should be clear that love is not examined here as an object of study in its own right; such an inquiry would require a separate analysis. In Lacan's work, love is approached from multiple angles and takes on different forms. Here it is used in a particular sense, as the point at which singular self-formation reaches its decisive articulation, thereby shedding light on how singularity takes shape in technological environments.

To grasp the distinctiveness of this position, it is useful to situate love within a longer philosophical and cultural tradition. Within this tradition, and in line with the analysis of desire developed here, love has often been understood in terms of completion and the expectation that it might provide it. In Plato's *Symposium*, this view of love finds vivid expression in Aristophanes' myth of originally whole beings. Round, self-sufficient and complete, these beings were split into two by the gods, leaving each half condemned to search for its lost counterpart. Ever since, each part longs to be reunited with the other, to overcome separation and restore an original unity. Love thus arises from division but is oriented toward its resolution, the recovery of wholeness through the encounter with the right other. This image continues to echo in the familiar idea of finding the one who makes us complete (Plato 1997).

At the same time, Plato's text already suggests that love is not reducible to harmony. Love does not simply restore unity; it interrupts the subject and unsettles its coordinates. This is not merely a thematic claim but is staged in the dialogue itself through a series of disruptions, indicating that love is located not in the achievement of balance but in the disturbance that interrupts it. This becomes clear at the level of the relation between lover and beloved. The lover seeks unity yet encounters no simple correspondence in the beloved. The beloved does not fully respond, does not coincide with what is expected and cannot be reduced to the role assigned to it. What emerges is not a relation of completion but one marked by a persistent asymmetry. This mismatch in the narrative is not incidental but constitutive of the relation itself.

Love thus confronts the subject with a failure of alignment that cannot be resolved. What sustains the relation is not the restoration of unity but the persistence of a gap between what is sought and what is encountered. This disturbance does not simply hinder love but belongs to its very movement.

Lacan's account radicalizes this insight by detaching it from any residual orientation toward completion. What in Plato still appears as a disturbance within a horizon of possible unity becomes, in Lacan, the very structure of the relation itself. Division is not a contingent loss but a structural condition. There is no lost unity to be recovered and no other who could complete the subject. The asymmetry between lover and beloved is no longer a failure within the relation but its defining feature. Love does not aim at overcoming this gap, nor does it presuppose that it could be resolved.

For Lacan, love, therefore, cannot be understood as the attainment, or even the deferred realization of wholeness, but as a way of relating to lack itself. This is captured in Lacan's formulation of love as "giving what you don't have" (Lacan 2015, 121). What is given is not a missing piece but the exposure of one's own incompleteness. To love is to approach the other without pretending to be whole, and without expecting the other to complete you. The other, in turn, is equally divided. What sustains the relation is not the hope of alignment but the persistence of a division that no encounter can resolve, and that love, precisely, does not aim to resolve.

This also clarifies the relation between love and desire. Desire, as developed throughout this study, is structured by lack and sustained by the movement around the object-cause. Love does not abolish this movement; it transforms its organization. The other is approached not as the bearer of what is missing but as a locus of desire that cannot be absorbed into one's own. What becomes possible is a relation no longer oriented toward the resolution of lack but sustained through it.

This entails a shift in how the other is encountered. The other cannot be fully known, predicted or rendered transparent, not because of insufficient information but because it is marked by the same irreducible division. Love begins where the other is no longer reduced to the coordinates of one's own fantasy but is encountered at the point where it exceeds them.

The encounter is therefore necessarily unsettling, as it disrupts and resists integration into the framework through which desire had been organized, confronting the subject with what cannot be anticipated, aligned or absorbed into its existing coordinates.

It is in this shift that the possibility of singularity appears. Love, in this sense, is the form this possibility takes. Singularity consists not in escaping desire but in assuming its structure without locating its resolution in the other. The relation is no longer organized around the expectation that the other will resolve one's lack, but is sustained without such an expectation.

This shift can be specified more precisely in terms of the movement from desire to drive. The metonymic movement of desire, characterized by a continuous slippage from one object to another, gives way to a movement that no longer seeks resolution in a new object but returns to the same place, circling around a structural void. In love, this takes a specific form: the partner is being approached not as an object that might finally fit but as the site in which the object-cause of desire is encountered. In this sense the subject comes to love *object a* it finds in the partner (Fink 2016, 102). What is sustained is not the promise of completion but the relation to lack itself, as that which continues to organize desire without ever being resolved.

From this perspective the account of love developed here clarifies what takes place in algorithmic environments and how openings for singularity may emerge within them. These environments organize the search for completion by structuring encounters as matters of compatibility, prediction and optimization. At the same time, by multiplying options and sustaining repetition, they render perceptible the instability of this very search. The promise that the right match will resolve division is not only maintained but continuously undermined by its own operation. What is exposed, in this way, is not simply the failure of particular matches but the persistence of a search that cannot be brought to completion.

What becomes possible under these conditions, however, is not a simple escape from the dynamics of the platform but a shift in how they are inhabited. This shift does not occur outside the processes of matching themselves. By pursuing matching to its limit, users may come to recognize the underlying pattern of neurotic search, the persistent hope that it will finally work. To go beyond neurosis, then, means not abandoning this search but coming to recognize its structure as such, treating it not as a path that might eventually succeed but as a movement organized around an expectation that cannot be fulfilled. It is this recognition, however fleeting, that can distance one from the dynamics of the platform. Love can mark such a moment, not because it resolves the structure but because it suspends, whether briefly or more enduringly, the expectation that it is to be resolved.

A more singular relation to algorithmic environments emerges when these are approached not as systems that reveal who one truly wants but as systems that stage and repeat one's own patterns of desire. Algorithmic suggestions, matches and patterns are no longer read as indicators of compatibility or as steps toward fulfillment but as elements that stage and repeat one's own position within desire. Desire does not come to an end but is sustained without the expectation of resolution or completion. The partner is no longer approached as the object that might finally fit but encountered as the locus of the object-cause of desire. What emerges between partners is therefore not a successful match but a disruption that unsettles the very coordinates of matching. In this sense, love does not introduce a relation outside these dynamics but marks a different way of inhabiting them: what is sustained is not the promise that lack will be overcome but a relation to it that no longer seeks its solution in the other.

Alongside this repositioning on the side of the subject, a further question arises concerning the environments themselves. If love names a way of relating that does not seek to resolve lack, it also clarifies what is at stake in the design of algorithmic environments: not the optimization of matching but whether the fantasy of alignment is continuously sustained or can be disrupted. The issue is therefore not simply how encounters are organized but whether they are staged as confirmations of compatibility or as situations in which noncoincidence can emerge and persist. This calls for forms of mediation that orient without stabilizing, guide without determining and structure encounters without closing the gap that animates desire. Platforms such as Tinder may create such openings to the extent that they make it perceptible that matches are not grounded in any necessary fit but are produced through the system's own operations, that they weaken the supposition that the system knows, interrupt cycles of optimization, and slow down the circulation of interchangeable options. What is at stake in such configurations is not improved matching but whether the encounter is immediately reabsorbed into the logic of compatibility or allowed to remain marked by the structural misalignment that love sustains.

Love, then, names neither a solution nor an achievement, but rather the point at which the demand for resolution is suspended. For this very reason, it also marks the limit of design: what defines love cannot be produced, predicted or secured as an outcome, since it depends on a disruption that no system can program in advance. Algorithmic environments may organize the conditions under which encounters occur, but they cannot determine how these encounters are taken up, nor whether they give rise to a relation that does not seek to resolve lack. In this sense, the structure of love is not only relevant to intimate relations, but reveals something more general about algorithmic environments as such: however far they extend the logic of optimization, prediction and alignment, they remain structurally unable to bring desire into coincidence with its object. Love makes this limit explicit: what sustains a relation is not the elimination of this gap but precisely the refusal to resolve it. It is here that singularity becomes possible, not as the product of design but as what may emerge where the demand for completion is suspended.

7 Epilogue

The Promise of Wholeness

A defining feature of contemporary culture is the enduring appeal of the promise of technology. In this respect, contemporary technologies do not stand apart from earlier historical constellations. Religions, ideologies and scientific worldviews have long claimed the capacity to overcome uncertainty, provide orientation and secure coherence for human existence. Technological promises can, at first glance, be understood as a continuation of this trajectory: yet another attempt to respond to the human condition by offering forms of meaning, stability and direction.

Upon closer inspection, however, a decisive shift becomes visible. What appears to be new is not the promise itself but its contemporary articulation. Unlike religions or ideologies, technological promises no longer present themselves as explicit responses to existential questions. They do not ask to be believed. Framed as advances in innovation, knowledge and capability, they appear as neutral instruments rather than as sources of meaning or salvation. Yet it is precisely in this displacement that their mode of operation changes. Technological promises do not announce themselves as responses to lack, even as they continue to engage it. Their appeal lies in the way they address desire indirectly, without requiring subjects to recognize that they are being existentially addressed at all. By presenting themselves as neutral means, they conceal the extent to which they shape how subjects seek existential orientation, coherence and recognition.

This concealment is further intensified by a transformation in the very form technology takes. Contemporary technologies operate primarily not as discrete instruments but as networked environments: layered constellations of data-driven infrastructures, computational operations and adaptive systems that continuously structure perception, interaction and experience. Within these technological environments, the address of desire becomes not only indirect but immersive and seamless. Rather than explicitly confronting subjects, they organize the conditions under which subjects come to recognize themselves, relate to others and articulate what they want. They shape how information appears, how choices are structured and how possibilities are encountered, all while maintaining the

DOI: 10.4324/9781042010912-7

appearance of neutrality and functionality. In doing so, they more effectively bypass the need for explicit ideological commitment and instead work through continuous engagement, interaction and adaptation.

In this shift from tools to environments, technological mediation becomes increasingly difficult to perceive. Technology no longer merely mediates but becomes a milieu; like a fish in water, subjects move within these environments and cannot do without them, without fully registering how they address their desire and shape the very horizon of their experience. It is through this indirect and often concealed mode of address, and through the immersive and seamless character of these technological environments, that technological promises gain their force and extend their reach. Technological promises do not merely offer technological solutions; by keeping the existential dimension hidden while nonetheless addressing it, they mobilize and relentlessly intensify our investment, drawing in vast resources and commitment, often against all odds.

This transformation intensifies and is normalized with the rise of algorithmic environments. Through continuous processes of data extraction, pattern recognition and feedback, these environments do more than structure visibility or anticipate action; they begin to present to subjects what they really seem to want. Preferences are inferred, choices are prestructured, and possibilities are offered in ways that feel tailored and self-evident. In this process, subjects encounter themselves in the form of predictions and recommendations that give the impression of mirroring their desires while in fact shaping them. The address operates here without declaration: it takes the form of recognition. What one takes to be one's own preference becomes increasingly inseparable from an environment that anticipates and formats it in advance.

Artificial intelligence, and especially generative AI, can now be understood as both a further refinement and a rupture within this trajectory. It builds on the same dynamics of prediction and anticipation yet transforms them by turning them into discursive and personalized interactions. It no longer merely presents back to subjects what they seem to want but actively participates in formulating and clarifying this wanting through sometimes very intimate dialogue. Where algorithmic environments suggest options or preferences, large language models engage subjects in ongoing exchanges in which desires are articulated, rephrased and refined in real time. In asking, responding and elaborating, they do not simply mirror what the subject wants but help bring it into language in a frictionless way, often before the subject could do so on its own. Their distinctive contribution lies not only in extending prediction but in turning it into a form of personal interaction: the subject increasingly encounters itself through responses that appear meaningful, coherent and tailored. In this way, AI intensifies the concealed address of desire by embedding it in dialogue, presenting the subject with an image of a desire that appears expressible, understandable and alignable while leaving the structural gap that sustains it intact.

Seen from this perspective, accounts that explain the expanding influence of technology primarily in terms of power, control or extraction remain incomplete. Zuboff has shown how data-driven systems anticipate and steer behavior, shaping markets and reinforcing asymmetries of power. Yet such accounts leave something essential unaddressed: the persistence and intensity of this investment, even when these dynamics are widely recognized. What the preceding chapters have made clear is that technological environments do not only operate upon subjects but resonate with the structure of desire itself, engaging subjects at the level where questions of orientation, recognition and coherence are at stake.

The analysis of Tinder has illustrated this dynamic in a particularly condensed form. As a paradigmatic technological environment, it does not merely facilitate encounters between individuals but structures the very field in which desire circulates. Through profiles, matches and continuous feedback, it stages the promise that the right encounter might finally resolve uncertainty, stabilize identity or deliver a form of completion. At the same time, it perpetuates the movement of desire by continuously deferring this promise. What appears as a sequence of individual choices is inseparable from an environment that anticipates, formats and returns desire in ways that both guide and sustain it. Tinder thus makes visible what often remains more concealed in other domains: that technological environments do not simply respond to desire but actively organize and intensify its circulation while maintaining the illusion that it might one day come to rest.

This existential approach also reframes how the question of resistance is to be understood. If the force of these environments lies not only in their capacity to monitor, steer and control but in the way they resonate with the structure of desire and subjectivity itself, then the response cannot be framed solely in terms of countering power or limiting influence. It must also involve a more reflective engagement with how subjects are and seek to be addressed, and how they position themselves in relation to this address. This shifts the focus from external opposition to a form of critical dialectics, in which the subject does not simply externalize and reject what is offered but interrogates the way in which it is drawn into it and engages with it. Such a shift becomes possible because this address never fully determines the subject, always leaving room for how it is taken up.

Seen in this light, the same processes that guide and structure desire also allow it to be rearticulated, confronting subjects with themselves in new ways. On the one hand, algorithmic environments can reinforce symbolic identifications or even reduce them to imaginary relations of comparison, visibility and recognition. The subject then becomes increasingly dependent on unstable norms, mirrors and shifting others. On the other hand, by loosening inherited and traditionally dominant frameworks, algorithmic environments can expose the subject to its own lack, bringing to the surface an instability they simultaneously attempt to conceal. The very mechanisms that bind subjects to patterns of anticipation and recognition may also create openings for interruption, reconfiguration and repositioning.

This has been described as the double bind of algorithmic environments. What was once organized around relatively stable Big Others gives way to a dispersed field of shifting small others, in which authority no longer presents itself as a unified point of reference but circulates across platforms, interfaces and algorithmic systems. The question "What do you want?" remains inseparable from the question "What does the Other want from me?" – yet it is less readily stabilized within a coherent symbolic order. As a result, this entanglement intensifies without any definitive point of anchoring. Precisely this combination of constant address and lack of anchoring deepens the subject's involvement: in search of orientation, it becomes more responsive to the fragmented order that addresses it. This condition can fully take hold of the subject, eroding any distance. Yet for that very reason it can also make such distance possible. The same disorientation that draws the subject in can enable it to take up the question of its desire and to negotiate its relation to what addresses it.

I have elaborated this double bind in more fine-grained terms through Lacan's clinical structures: psychosis, perversion, neurosis and what lies beyond them. To render these less clinical, I have translated them into figures: the absorbed, the pleaser, the seeker and the possibility of singular formation. These figures, as I have reframed them, designate ways of relating to the structural lack that technological environments both conceal and mobilize. The absorbed dissolves into the technological coordinates provided, relinquishing any distance to what is anticipated. The pleaser aligns with the perceived expectations of the algorithmic Other, seeking recognition within the circuits that address it. The seeker remains caught in the endless pursuit of a fitting object, moving from one promise to the next. Singular formation, by contrast, no longer organizes itself around the fantasy of wholeness but takes up lack by shifting from desire to drive. In doing so the subject can, if only momentarily, remain with its lack by encountering the object in its function as cause, as in the structure of love. These positions are not external to technological environments but emerge within them as distinct ways of inhabiting their address.

Within this framework the Lacanian account of desire clarifies why subjects are both less and more than their data (Aydin and Possati 2025). They are "less" than their data insofar as their identities depend on symbolic and technological infrastructures that render them coherent, legible and socially viable, yet they are also paradoxically "more" than their data because they inevitably fail to coincide with the representations these systems produce.

This noncoincidence is not new; it has always marked the relation between subject and symbolic form. What is specific to algorithmic environments, however, is how this gap is continuously produced and returned. Through ongoing processes of data capture, prediction and feedback, subjects are repeatedly confronted with representations that claim to anticipate and fix who they are and what they want. Yet precisely through this continuous return, and the need to constantly recalibrate oneself in response to shifting and unstable Big Others, the impossibility of full coincidence becomes harder to ignore. The subject encounters itself as both captured and missed by its data. This is the double bind at the level of data: the same representations that seek to stabilize and anticipate the subject also expose the gap through which it fails to be fully captured by them. Under these conditions, both regression and the emergence of singular forms become possible.

However, this account gives rise to an important question, one that initially seems to challenge its premises. If the gap that sustains desire can, under certain conditions, become productive, it may seem less evident that desire can be understood exclusively in terms of lack. What comes into view is not only a relation to what is missing but also a dynamic in which new positions and possibilities are generated. In contemporary technological environments, the proliferation of options, connections and trajectories suggests a field in which desire no longer appears anchored in lack, but moves across an expanding landscape of possibilities. Under these conditions, the subject appears not only as marked by lack and division but also as capable of multiplicity, excess and a certain generative richness. This intuition finds resonance in a range of philosophical approaches. Gilles Deleuze and Félix Guattari, for instance, emphasize the productive and connective dimensions of desire. Friedrich Nietzsche understands willing in terms of life's excess and affirmation. Georges Bataille, in turn, foregrounds its dimension of expenditure and surplus beyond utility.

Yet this appearance misleads. What presents itself as abundance does not displace lack; the multiplication of possibilities does not overcome noncoincidence but extends and intensifies it. The point is not that multiplicity, excess or expenditure are illusory or unreal, but that they cannot arise without lack. In this sense, accounts that foreground productivity and excess do not move beyond lack but rely on it. Desire moves only because it never fully coincides with itself. It is precisely this noncoincidence that enables multiplicity, differentiation and proliferation. Without this gap there would be no excess, no creativity, no richness of possibilities. Abundance does not replace lack; it depends on it and gives it form.

What this study has sought to show, therefore, is not that lack is something to be corrected, resolved or filled. Neither older dogmatic systems nor contemporary technological environments eliminate this lack; instead, they tend to conceal it by creating the impression that it can be resolved, even as they continue to rely on it. What emerges in contemporary technological environments is a far-reaching attempt to organize and anticipate this relation to lack, an ongoing engineering of desire that structures how subjects encounter, articulate and pursue what they take themselves to want. This engineering does not resolve desire but reconfigures its conditions: it redistributes how objects appear, how trajectories unfold, and how recognition is sought while leaving intact the structural noncoincidence through which desire persists. The multiplication of options, matches, recommendations and responses does not bring desire to rest but sustains its movement by continuously rearticulating what might count as its object.

What is at stake, then, is not whether desire can be brought to completion but how subjects position themselves in relation to these processes. The openness that constitutes the subject is easily taken as something that could be filled by a particular object, whether promised by religion, ideology or technology. In doing so, what cannot be resolved is repeatedly translated into something that appears attainable, sustaining the movement of desire while obscuring its structure. To take up the self as lack is to move through this misrecognition and the fantasy of wholeness that sustains it, without the illusion that one could ever fully escape it. It is here that the possibility of singularity emerges, not as the resolution of desire but as a way of inhabiting it without deferring its question. Understood as its singular aim, desire comes into view at the moment when the question "What do I want" is no longer deferred, outsourced or silently answered in advance but taken up as mine, in and through the very environments that seek to organize and engineer it.

Bibliography

Abi-Rached, J. M., and N. Rose. 2010a. *Neuro: The New Brain Sciences and the Management of the Mind*. Princeton, NJ: Princeton University Press.

Abi-Rached, J. M., and N. Rose. 2010b. "The Human Brain Project: From Mapping to Moral Reasoning." *Neuron* 67 (3): 422–435.

Anscombe, G. E. M. 2000. *Intention*. Cambridge, MA: Harvard University Press.

Arpaly, N., and T. Schroeder. 2014. *In Praise of Desire*. Oxford: Oxford University Press.

Aydin, C. 2007. "Nietzsche on Reality as Will to Power: Toward an 'Organization-Struggle Model.'" *Journal of Nietzsche Studies* 33: 25–48.

Aydin, C. 2017. "The Posthuman as Hollow Idol: A Nietzschean Critique of Human Enhancement." *Journal of Medicine and Philosophy* 42 (3): 304–327.

Aydin, C. 2021. *Extimate Technology: Self-Formation in a Technological World*. New York: Routledge.

Aydin, C., M. González-Woge, and P.-P. Verbeek. 2019. "Technological Environmentality: Conceptualizing Technology as a Mediating Milieu." *Philosophy and Technology* 32 (2): 321–338.

Aydin, C., and L. Possati. 2025. "Less and More than Data: A Lacanian Inquiry into Self-Formation in the Age of Data Mining." *AI & Society* 40: 6123–6134.

Baker, S. A., L. J. Krieger, and T. E. LeRoy. 2019. "Selfie-Posting Behaviors and Personality: Who Posts Selfies and Why?" *Personality and Individual Differences* 133: 279–284.

Bandinelli, C., and J. Johanssen. 2022. "Algorithmic Intimacy: The Platformization of Romantic Desire." *Communication and Critical/Cultural Studies* 19 (1): 1–17.

Bandhu, D., M. M. Mohan, N. A. P. Nittala, P. Jadhav, A. Bhadauria, and K. K. Saxena. 2024. "Theories of Motivation: A Comprehensive Analysis of Human Behavior Drivers." *Acta Psychologica* 244: 104177. https://doi.org/10.1016/j.actpsy.2024.104177

Banet-Weiser, S. 2018. *Empowered: Popular Feminism and Popular Misogyny*. Durham, NC: Duke University Press.

Barrada, J. R., and Á. Castro. 2020. "Tinder Users: Sociodemographic, Psychological, and Psychosexual Characteristics." *International Journal of Environmental Research and Public Health* 17 (21): 8047.

Bauman, Z. 2000. *Liquid Modernity*. Cambridge: Polity Press.

Beerends, S., N. Gertz, and C. Aydin. 2026. "AI and the Machinization of Humans: An Escape from the Burdens of Existence." *AI and Ethics* 6: 301. https://doi.org/10.1007/s43681-026-01126-y

Bell, B. T., R. Lawton, and H. Dittmar. 2016. "'I Always Look Skinnier in the Mirror': Appearance Comparisons and Body Image in Young Adult Women." *Body Image* 16: 107–113.

Berridge, K. C., and M. L. Kringelbach. 2015. "Pleasure Systems in the Brain." *Neuron* 86 (3): 646–664.

Besley, T. 2008. *Subjectivity & Truth: Foucault, Education, and the Culture of Self*. New York: Peter Lang.

Bleize, D. N. M., A. van Stekelenburg, and S. L. Tamboer. 2023. "The Association Between Mobile Dating App Use and Relationship Status Satisfaction: A Survey Study." *Mobile Media & Communication* 11 (3): 456–475.

Bommasani, R., Creel, K. A., Kumar, A., Jurafsky, D., and Liang, P. S. 2022. "Picking on the Same Person: Does Algorithmic Monoculture Lead to Outcome Homogenization?" *Advances in Neural Information Processing Systems*, 35: 3663–3678.

Bown, A. 2015. *Enjoying It: Candy Cruch and Capitalism*. Winchester: Zero Books.

Braunstein, N. 2003. "Desire and Jouissance in the Teachings of Lacan." In *Lacan and the New Wave in American Psychoanalysis*, edited by B. Fink, 45–68. New York: Other Press.

Brook, A. 2006. *A Unified Theory of Mind and Brain*. Cambridge: Cambridge University Press.

Brown, Z., and M. Tiggemann. 2016. "Attractive Celebrity and Peer Images on Instagram: Effect on Women's Mood and Body Image." *Body Image* 19: 37–43.

Budennyy, S. A., V. D. Lazarev, N. N. Zakharenko, A. N. Korovin, O. A. Plosskaya, D. V. E. Dimitrov, and L. E. E. Zhukov. 2022. "Eco2AI: Carbon Emissions Tracking of Machine Learning Models as the First Step Towards Sustainable AI." *Doklady Mathematics* 106 (Suppl. 1): S118–S128.

Carpenter, C. J., and B. McEwan. 2016. "The Players of Micro-Dating: Individual and Social Characteristics of Tinder Users." *Computers in Human Behavior* 55: 117–122.

Carter, J. 2012. "Young People's Relationships: Learning and Practising Intimacy." *Sociological Review* 60 (3): 611–630.

Carter, J. 2017. "Why Marry? The Role of Tradition in Women's Marital Aspirations." *Sociological Research Online* 22 (1): 1–17.

Carter, J., and S. Duncan. 2016. "Wedding Paradoxes: Individualized Conformity and the 'Perfect Day'." *Sociological Review* 65 (1): 3–20.

Chaumon, F. 2004. *The Unconscious and the Real: Lacanian Theory and Clinical Practice*. London: Karnac Books.

Cheney-Lippold, J. 2017. *We Are Data: Algorithms and the Making of Our Digital Selves*. New York: NYU Press.

Clavreul, J. 1980. *The Ethics of Psychoanalysis*. London: Free Association Books.

Colbrook, M. J., V. Antun, and A. C. Hansen. 2022. "The Difficulty of Computing Stable and Accurate Neural Networks: On the Barriers of Deep Learning and Smale's 18th Problem." *Proceedings of the National Academy of Sciences* 119 (12): e2107151119.

ConsumerAffairs. 2026. "Tinder Reviews." Accessed January 7, 2026. https://www.consumeraffairs.com/dating_services/tinder.html

Crawford, K. 2021. *The Atlas of AI: Power, Politics, and the Planetary Costs of Artificial Intelligence*. New Haven, CT: Yale University Press.

Davidson, D. 1980. *Essays on Actions and Events*. Oxford: Clarendon Press.

Davis, W. A. 1984. "A Causal Theory of Intending." *American Philosophical Quarterly* 21 (1): 43–54.

De Mul, J. 2004. *The Tragedy of Finitude: Dilthey's Hermeneutics of Life*. New Haven, CT: Yale University Press.

De Mul, J. 2015. "Database Identity: Personal and Cultural Identity in the Age of Global Datafication." In *25 Years of Privacy Law: Time for a Data Revolution?* edited by B. van den Berg and S. van der Hof, 103–116. The Hague: Asser Press.

Deleuze, G., and F. Guattari. 1972. *Anti-Oedipus: Capitalism and Schizophrenia*. Translated by R. Hurley, M. Seem, and H. R. Lane. Minneapolis: University of Minnesota Press.

Elliott, A. 2015. *Psychoanalytic Theory: An Introduction*. London: Palgrave Macmillan.

Erevik, E. K., S. Pallesen, M. M. Andreassen, and S. S. Torsheim. 2020. "Tinder Use and Romantic Relationship Formations: A Large-Scale Longitudinal Study." *Frontiers in Psychology* 11: 1757.

Eubanks, V. 2018. *Automating Inequality: How High-Tech Tools Profile, Police, and Punish the Poor*. New York: St. Martin's Press.

Evans, D. 1996. *An Introductory Dictionary of Lacanian Psychoanalysis*. London: Routledge.

Fenichel, O. 1945. *The Psychoanalytic Theory of Neurosis*. New York: W. W. Norton & Company.

Fink, B. 1997. *The Lacanian Subject: Between Language and Jouissance*. Princeton, NJ: Princeton University Press.

Fink, B. 1999. *A Clinical Introduction to Lacanian Psychoanalysis: Theory and Technique*. Cambridge, MA: Harvard University Press.

Fink, B. 2016. *Lacan on Love: An Exploration of Lacan's Seminar VIII, Transference*. Cambridge: Polity Press.

Flisfeder, M. 2021. *Algorithmic Desire: Toward a New Structuralist Theory of Social Media*. Evanston: Northwestern University Press.

Floridi, L. 2021. *The Logic of Information: A Theory of Philosophy as Conceptual Design*. Oxford: Oxford University Press.

Foucault, M. 1977. *Discipline and Punish: The Birth of the Prison*. Translated by A. Sheridan. New York: Pantheon Books.

Fox, J., and M. C. Rooney. 2015. "The Dark Triad and Trait Self-Objectification as Predictors of Men's Use and Self-Presentation Behaviors on Social Networking Sites." *Personality and Individual Differences* 76: 161–165.

Frankfurt, H. G. 1971. "Freedom of the Will and the Concept of a Person." *The Journal of Philosophy* 68 (1): 5–20.

Frankfurt, H. G. 1999. *Necessity, Volition, and Love*. Cambridge: Cambridge University Press.

Freud, S. 1981. *The Standard Edition of the Complete Psychological Works of Sigmund Freud*. London: Vintage.

Furman, A. C., and S. T. Levy, eds. 2003. *Influential Papers from the 1950s*. London: Karnac.

Gemes, K. 2009. "Freud and Nietzsche on Sublimation." *Journal of Nietzsche Studies* 38 (1): 38–59.

Gill, R. 2007. *Gender and the Media*. Cambridge: Polity Press.

Gillespie, T. 2014. "The Relevance of Algorithms." In *Media Technologies: Essays on Communication, Materiality, and Society*, edited by T. Gillespie, P. J. Boczkowski, and K. A. Foot, 167–194. Cambridge, MA: MIT Press.

Grosman, J., and T. Reigeluth. 2019. "Perspectives on Algorithmic Normativities: Engineers, Objects, Activities." *Big Data & Society* 6 (2): 1–12.

Han, J., M. Kamber, and J. Pei. 2022. *Data Mining: Concepts and Techniques*. San Francisco: Morgan Kaufmann.

Hanna, E., L. M. Ward, R. C. Seabrook, M. Jerald, L. Reed, S. Giaccardi, and J. R. Lippman. 2017. "Contributions of Social Comparison and Self-Objectification in Mediating Associations Between Facebook Use and Emergent Adults' Psychological Well-Being." *Cyberpsychology, Behavior, and Social Networking* 20 (3): 172–179.

Hawes, T., M. J. Zimmer-Gembeck, and S. M. Campbell. 2020. "Unique Associations of Social Media Use and Online Appearance Preoccupation with Depression, Anxiety, and Appearance Rejection Sensitivity." *Body Image* 33: 66–76.

Hegel, G. W. F. 2018. *The Phenomenology of Spirit*. Translated by Terry Pinkard. Cambridge: Cambridge University Press.

Heino, R. D., N. B. Ellison, and J. L. Gibbs. 2010. "Relationshopping: Investigating the Market Metaphor in Online Dating." *Journal of Social and Personal Relationships* 27 (4): 427–447.

Her, Y. C., and E. Timmermans. 2020. "Tinder Blue, Mental Flu? Exploring the Associations Between Tinder Use and Well-Being." *Information, Communication & Society* 24 (9): 1303–1319.

Hobbs, M., S. Owen, and L. Gerber. 2017. "Liquid Love? Dating Apps, Sex, Relationships and the Digital Transformation of Intimacy." *Journal of Sociology* 53 (2): 271–284.

Holtzhausen, N., K. Fitzgerald, I. Thakur, J. Ashley, M. Rolfe, and S. W. Pit. 2020. "Swipe-Based Dating Applications Use and Its Association with Mental Health Outcomes: A Cross-Sectional Study." *BMC Psychology* 8 (1): 1–12.

Homer, S. 2005. *Jacques Lacan*. London: Routledge.

Hulse, D., C. Read, and T. Schroeder. 2004. "The Impossibility of Conscious Desire." *American Philosophical Quarterly* 41 (1): 73–80.

Illouz, E. 1997. *Consuming the Romantic Utopia: Love and the Cultural Contradictions of Capitalism*. Berkeley: University of California Press.

Illouz, E. 2007. *Cold Intimacies: The Making of Emotional Capitalism*. Cambridge: Polity Press.

Illouz, E. 2012. *Why Love Hurts: A Sociological Explanation*. Cambridge: Polity Press.

Illouz, E. 2017. "Toward a Post-Normative Critique of Emotional Authenticity: Capitalism, Consumption and Authenticity." *Theory, Culture & Society* 34 (1): 3–28.

Illouz, E. 2022. *The End of Love: A Sociology of Negative Relations*. Oxford: Oxford University Press.

Illouz, E., and D. M. Kotliar. 2022. "Capitalist Subjectivity, Tinder, and the Emotionalization of the Web." In R. Llamas and R. Belk (Eds.), *The Routledge Handbook of Digital Consumption* (2nd ed.), 229–240. London: Routledge.

Iqbal, M. 2025. "Tinder Statistics." *Business of Apps*. https://www.businessofapps.com/data/tinder-statistics/

Jackson, L. 2021. "Shoshana Zuboff Explains Why You Should Care About Privacy." *The New York Times*, May 21, 2021. https://www.nytimes.com/2021/05/21/technology/shoshana-zuboff-apple-google-privacy.html

Jamieson, L. 1998. *Intimacy: Personal Relationships in Modern Societies*. Cambridge: Polity Press.

Julien, P. 1990. *Jacques Lacan's Return to Freud: The Real, the Symbolic, and the Imaginary*. New York: NYU Press.

Katz, E., J. G. Blumler, and M. Gurevitch. 1973. "Uses and Gratifications Research." *Public Opinion Quarterly* 37 (4): 509–523.

Kavenna, J. 2019. "Shoshana Zuboff: 'Surveillance Capitalism Is an Assault on Human Autonomy.'" *The Guardian*, October 4, 2019. https://www.theguardian.com/books/2019/oct/04/shoshana-zuboff-surveillance-capitalism-assault-human-automomy-digital-privacy

Kemberg, O. F. 2020. "Malignant Narcissism and Large Group Regression." *The Psychoanalytic Quarterly 89* (1): 1–24.

Lacan, J. 1962. *The Seminar of Jacques Lacan, Book IX: Identification*. Unpublished manuscript, session of June 13, 1962.

Lacan, J. 1977. *The Seminar of Jacques Lacan, Book XI: The Four Fundamental Concepts of Psychoanalysis*. New York: W. W. Norton & Company.

Lacan, J. 1988. *The Seminar of Jacques Lacan, Book II: The Ego in Freud's Theory and in the Technique of Psychoanalysis, 1954–1955*. Translated by S. Tomaselli. Cambridge: Cambridge University Press.

Lacan, J. 1991. *The Seminar of Jacques Lacan, Book II: The Ego in Freud's Theory and in the Technique of Psychoanalysis, 1954–1955*. Edited by J.-A. Miller. Translated by S. Tomaselli. New York: W. W. Norton & Company.

Lacan, J. 1992. *The Seminar of Jacques Lacan, Book VII: The Ethics of Psychoanalysis, 1959–1960*. London: Routledge.
Lacan, J. 1997. *The Seminar of Jacques Lacan, Book III: The Psychoses, 1955–1956*. New York: W. W. Norton & Company.
Lacan, J. 1998. *The Seminar of Jacques Lacan, Book XX: Encore, 1972–1973*. New York: W. W. Norton & Company.
Lacan, J. 2005. *The Sinthome: The Seminar of Jacques Lacan, Book XXIII, 1975–1976*. Translated by A. R. Price. Cambridge: Polity Press.
Lacan, J. 2006. *Écrits: The First Complete Edition in English*. Translated by B. Fink. New York: W. W. Norton & Company.
Lacan, J. 2007. *The Seminar of Jacques Lacan, Book XVII: The Other Side of Psychoanalysis, 1969–1970*. Edited by R. Grigg. New York: W. W. Norton.
Lacan, J. 2014. *The Seminar of Jacques Lacan, Book X: Anxiety, 1962–1963*. Translated by A. R. Price. Cambridge: Polity Press.
Lacan, J. 2015. *The Seminar of Jacques Lacan, Book VIII: Transference, 1960–1961*. Translated by B. Fink. Cambridge: Polity Press.
Lacan, J. 2016. *My Teaching*. Translated by B. Fink. London: W. W. Norton & Company.
Lacan, J. 2017. *The Seminar of Jacques Lacan, Book V: Formations of the Unconscious, 1957–1958*. Cambridge: Polity Press.
LaGrandeur, K. 2024. "The Consequences of AI Hype." *AI and Ethics* 4 (3): 653–656.
Laplanche, J., and J. B. Pontalis. 1973. *The Language of Psycho-Analysis*. Translated by D. Nicholson-Smith. New York: W. W. Norton & Company.
Lasch, C. 1979. *The Culture of Narcissism: American Life in an Age of Diminishing Expectations*. New York: W. W. Norton & Company.
Latham, N. 2006. "Desires, Dispositions, and the Explanation of Action." *Philosophical Studies* 130 (3): 565–595.
Lavidge, R. J., and G. A. Steiner. 1961. "A Model for Predictive Measurements of Advertising Effectiveness." *Journal of Marketing* 25 (6): 59–62.
Levine, S. Z. 2008. *Lacan Reframed: Interpreting Key Thinkers for the Arts*. London: I.B. Tauris.
Lewis, D. 1972. "Psychophysical and Theoretical Identifications." *Australasian Journal of Philosophy* 50 (3): 249–258.
Lolli, F. 2022. *Vivere la pulsione: Saggio sulla soddisfazione in psicoanalisi*. Napoli: Ortothes.
Loose, R. 2023. *Lacan on Addiction*. London: Routledge.
Lovallo, D., and A. Webb. 2011. "Nudging the World toward Smarter Public Policy: An Interview with Richard Thaler." *McKinsey Quarterly*, June 1, 2011. https://www.mckinsey.com/industries/public-sector/our-insights/nudging-the-world-toward-smarter-public-policy-an-interview-with-richard-thaler
Maggiori, E. 2023. *Smart Until It's Dumb: Why Artificial Intelligence Keeps Making Epic Mistakes (and Why the AI Bubble Will Burst)*. London: Applied Maths Limited.

Malaspina, C. 2018. *An Epistemology of Noise*. London: Bloomsbury Academic.

Malenka, R. C., E. J. Nestler, and S. E. Hyman. 2009. *Molecular Neuropharmacology: A Foundation for Clinical Neuroscience*. 2nd ed. New York: McGraw-Hill Medical.

Marcus, G. 2018. "Deep Learning: A Critical Appraisal." *arXiv preprint arXiv:1801.00631*. https://arxiv.org/pdf/1801.00631

Marcus, G. 2025. "The Most Underreported and Important Story in AI Right Now Is That Pure Scaling Has Failed to Produce AGI." *Fortune*, February 19, 2025. https://fortune.com/2025/02/19/generative-ai-scaling-agi-deep-learning/

Markelius, A., C. Wright, J. Kuiper, N. Delille, and Y. T. Kuo. 2024. "The Mechanisms of AI Hype and Its Planetary and Social Costs." *AI and Ethics* 4 (3): 727–742.

Marks, J. 1986. "A Theory of Emotion." *Philosophical Studies* 49 (3): 341–357.

Martínez, G., L. Watson, P. Reviriego, J. A. Hernández, M. Juarez, and R. Sarkar. 2023. "Combining Generative Artificial Intelligence (AI) and the Internet: Heading towards Evolution or Degradation?" *arXiv preprint*, February 17. https://doi.org/10.48550/arXiv.2303.01255

Matviyenko, S. 2015. "The Imaginary of the Algorithm." *Digital Culture & Society* 1 (1): 89–104.

McDaniel, K., and B. Bradley. 2008. "Desires." *Mind* 117 (466): 267–302.

McGowan, T. 2016. *Capitalism and Desire: The Psychic Cost of Free Markets*. New York: Columbia University Press.

McGowan, T. 2024. *Embracing Alienation: Why We Shouldn't Try to Find Ourselves*. London: Repeater Books.

McGowan, T. *Why Theory*. Podcast by Todd McGowan and Ryan Engley. https://whytheorypodcast.libsyn.com

Meier, E. P., and J. Gray. 2014. "Facebook Photo Activity Associated with Body Image Disturbance in Adolescent Girls." *Cyberpsychology, Behavior, and Social Networking* 17 (4): 199–206.

Miller, J.-A. 2011. "Being Is Desire." Lacan.com, May 11, 2011. https://www.lacan.com/symptom/being-is-desire-jacques-alain-miller/

Mooij, A. 2018. *Lacan and Cassirer: An Essay on Symbolisation*. Leiden: Brill | Rodopi.

Morillo, C. R. 1990. "The Reward Event and Motivation." *The Journal of Philosophy* 87 (4): 169–186.

Moyaert, P. 2011. "Wat ons bindt aan een werkelijkheid die vereenzaamt. Hoe Lacan nadenkt over ethiek." *Ethische Perspectieven* 21 (3): 230–257.

Munn, L. 2023. "The Uselessness of AI Ethics." *AI and Ethics 3* (3): 869–877.

Murray, H. A. 1938. *Explorations in Personality*. New York: Oxford University Press.

Nietzsche, F. 2002. *Beyond Good and Evil*. Edited by R. P. Horstmann and J. Norman. Cambridge: Cambridge University Press.

Noble, S. U. 2018. *Algorithms of Oppression: How Search Engines Reinforce Racism*. New York: New York University Press.

Oddie, G. 2005. *Value, Reality, and Desire*. Oxford: Clarendon Press.

Paranjpe, A. C. 2022. *Yoga and Psychoanalysis: Perspectives on the Psychology of Regression*. New York: Routledge.

Pasquinelli, M. 2023. *The Eye of the Master: A Social History of Artificial Intelligence*. London: Verso.

Plato. 1997. *The Symposium*. Translated by C. Gill. London: Penguin Classics.

Quora. 2026. "What Has Been Your Best Tinder Experience When Seeking Serious Dating?" Accessed February 25, 2026. https://www.quora.com/What-has-been-your-best-Tinder-experience-when-seeking-serious-dating

Rambatan, B., and J. Johanssen. 2021. *Fantasy, Online Misogyny and the Manosphere: Male Bodies of Dis/Inhibition*. London: Routledge.

Ranzini, G., and C. Lutz. 2017. "Love at First Swipe? Explaining Tinder Self-Presentation and Motives." *Mobile Media & Communication* 5 (1): 80–101.

Recalcati, M. 2023. "For a Clinical Theory of the Institution." In *Capitalism and the New Political Unconscious*, edited by F. Vighi and R. Panattoni, 23–35. London: Bloomsbury Academic.

Reddit. 2026. "The Absolute State of Dating Apps in 2024." *r/assholedesign*. Accessed February 25, 2026. https://www.reddit.com/r/assholedesign/comments/1bvgjwg/the_absolute_state_of_dating_apps_in_2024/

Romele, A. 2019. *Digital Hermeneutics: Philosophical Investigations in New Media and Technologies*. London: Routledge.

Rose, N. 2007. *The Politics of Life Itself: Biomedicine, Power, and Subjectivity in the Twenty-First Century*. Princeton, NJ: Princeton University Press.

Rosenfeld, M. J. 2018. "Are Tinder and Dating Apps Changing Dating and Mating in the USA?" In *Families and Technology*, edited by J. Van Hook, S. McHale, and V. King, 103–117. Cham: Springer.

Ruggiero, T. E. 2000. "Uses and Gratifications Theory in the 21st Century." *Mass Communication & Society* 3 (1): 3–37.

Ruti, M. 2012. *The Singularity of Being: Lacan and the Immortal Within*. New York: Fordham University Press.

Ryan, R. M., A. J. Bradshaw, and E. L. Deci. 2019. "A History of Human Motivation Theories." *Self-Determination Theory Research Papers*. https://selfdeterminationtheory.org/wp-content/uploads/2019/07/2019_RyanBradshawDeci_HistoryOfMotivationTheories.pdf

Saiphoo, A. N., and Z. Vahedi. 2019. "A Meta-Analytic Review of the Relationship Between Social Media Use and Body Image Disturbance." *Computers in Human Behavior* 101: 259–275.

Sands, S., and J. J. Ratey. 2023. "The Concept of Noise." *Angelaki* 28 (3): 16–24.

Sartre, J.-P. 2003. *Being and Nothingness*. Translated by H. E. Barnes. New York: Washington Square Press.

Scanlon, T. M. 1998. *What We Owe to Each Other*. Cambridge, MA: Harvard University Press.

Schroeder, T. 2004. *Three Faces of Desire*. New York: Oxford University Press.

Schroeder, T. 2009. "Desire." *Stanford Encyclopedia of Philosophy*. https://plato.stanford.edu/entries/desire/

Schueler, G. F. 1995. *Desire: Its Role in Practical Reason and the Explanation of Action*. Cambridge, MA: MIT Press.

Seaver, F. R. 2019. "*A Comparison of Static, Dynamic, and Machine Learning Models in Predicting the Financial Distress of Chinese Firms.*" *Proceedings of the 24th International Conference on Methods and Models in Automation and Robotics*, 1–6.

Sharabi, L. L., and E. Dorrance-Hall. 2024. "The Online Dating Effect: Where a Couple Meets Predicts the Quality of Their Marriage." *Computers in Human Behavior* 150: 107973.

Shaw, G. B. 1903. *Man and Superman*. London: Archibald Constable.

Smart, C. 2007. *Personal Life: New Directions in Sociological Thinking*. Cambridge: Polity Press.

Smith, M. 1987. "The Humean Theory of Motivation." *Mind* 96 (381): 36–61.

Smith, M. 1994. *The Moral Problem*. Oxford: Blackwell.

Sophocles. 1984. *The Three Theban Plays*. Translated by Robert Fagles. Harmondsworth: Penguin.

Stampe, D. W. 1986. "Defining Desire." In *The Ways of Desire: New Essays in Philosophical Psychology on the Concept of Wanting*, edited by J. Marks, 159–178. Chicago, IL: Precedent Publishing.

Stampe, P. W. J. 1987. "The Authority of Desire." *The Philosophical Review* 96 (3): 335–381.

Stephens-Davidowitz, S. 2017. *Everybody Lies: Big Data, New Data, and What the Internet Can Tell Us About Who We Really Are*. New York: HarperCollins.

Strange, M. 2024. "Three Different Types of AI Hype in Healthcare." *AI and Ethics* 4 (3): 833–840.

Strübel, J. 2023. "The Most Swipeable You: Experiences and Self-Perception of Tinder Users." *The Journal of American Culture* 46 (1): 44–54.

Strübel, J., and T. A. Petrie. 2017. "Love Me Tinder: Body Image and Psychosocial Functioning Among Men and Women." *Body Image* 21: 34–38.

Sumter, S. R., L. Vandenbosch, and L. Ligtenberg. 2017. "Love Me Tinder: Untangling Emerging Adults' Motivations for Using the Dating Application Tinder." *Telematics and Informatics* 34 (1): 67–78.

Tanner, M., and M. Huggins. 2018. "Why Swipe Right? Women's Motivation for Using Mobile Dating Applications Such as Tinder." *Journal of Business Diversity* 18 (2): 78–87.

Thaler, R. H., and C. R. Sunstein. 2003. "Libertarian Paternalism." *American Economic Review* 93 (2): 175–179.

Thaler, R. H., and C. R. Sunstein. 2008. *Nudge: Improving Decisions About Health, Wealth, and Happiness*. New Haven, CT: Yale University Press.

Thaler, R. H., and C. R. Sunstein. 2021. *Nudge: The Final Edition*. New York: Penguin Books.

The Economist. 2024. "What Happened to the Artificial-Intelligence Revolution? So Far the Technology Has Had Almost No Economic Impact." July 2, 2024. https://www.economist.com/finance-and-economics/2024/07/02/what-happened-to-the-artificial-intelligence-revolution

Tinder. 2026. "Tinder." Accessed February 25, 2026. https://www.tinder.com

Tomšič, S. 2015. *The Capitalist Unconscious: Marx and Lacan*. London: Verso.

Trekels, J., M. L. Ward, and S. Eggermont. 2018. "I 'Like' the Way You Look: How Appearance-Focused and Overall Facebook Use Contribute to Adolescents' Self-Sexualization." *Computers in Human Behavior* 81: 198–208.

Trustpilot. 2026. "Tinder Reviews." Accessed February 25, 2026. https://www.trustpilot.com/review/tinder.com?page=3

Turkle, S. 2011. *Evocative Objects: Things We Think With*. Cambridge, MA: MIT Press.

Turkle, S. 2016. *Reclaiming Conversation: The Power of Talk in a Digital Age*. New York: Penguin.

Turkle, S. 2017. *Alone Together*. New York: Basic Books.

Vadas, M. 1984. "Affective and Non-Affective Desire." *Philosophical Studies* 45 (2): 273–295.

Van Dijck, J. 2014. "Datafication, Dataism, and Dataveillance: Big Data Between Scientific Paradigm and Ideology." *Surveillance & Society* 12 (2): 197–208.

Van Haute, P. 2001. *Against Adaptation: Lacan's Subversion of the Subject*. New York: Other Press.

Van Hooff, J. H. 2013. "Modern Couples? Continuity and Change in Heterosexual Relationships." *Sociological Research Online* 18 (4): 1–23.

Van Hooff, J. H. 2017. "An Everyday Affair: Deciphering the Sociological Significance of Women's Attitudes Towards Infidelity." *Sociological Review* 65 (4): 850–866.

Vanheule, S. 2011. *The Subject of Psychosis: A Lacanian Perspective*. London: Palgrave Macmillan.

Vera Cruz, G., E. Aboujaoude, L. Rochat, F. Bianchi-Demichelli, and Y. Khazaal. 2023. "Finding Intimacy Online: A Machine Learning Analysis of Predictors of Success." *Cyberpsychology, Behavior, and Social Networking* 26 (8): 604–612.

Von Neumann, J., and O. Morgenstern. 1944. *Theory of Games and Economic Behavior*. Princeton, NJ: Princeton University Press.

Vox. 2020. "How Tinder Changed the Game of Dating Forever." https://www.vox.com

Ward, L. M., R. C. Seabrook, A. Manago, and L. Reed. 2016. "Contributions of Diverse Media to Self-Sexualization Among Undergraduate Women and Men." *Sex Roles* 74: 112–123.

Weinmann, M., C. Schneider, and J. vom Brocke. 2016a. "Digital Nudging." *Business & Information Systems Engineering* 58 (6): 433–436.

Weinmann, M., C. Schneider, and J. vom Brocke. 2016b. *Digital Nudging: Guiding Online Users' Decisions*. Springer. https://doi.org/10.1007/s12599-016-0453-1

Westerstrand, S., R. Westerstrand, and J. Koskinen. 2024. "Talking Existential Risk into Being: A Habermasian Critical Discourse Perspective to AI Hype." *AI and Ethics* 4 (3): 713–726.

Wilde, O. 1892. *Lady Windermere's Fan*. London: Elkin Mathews and John Lane.

Wise, J. 2023. Tinder Statistics 2023: How Many People Use Tinder? *EarthWeb*. https://earthweb.com/tinder-statistics/

Witten, I. H., E. Frank, M. A. Hall, and C. Pal. 2016. *Data Mining: Practical Machine Learning Tools and Techniques*. 4th ed. New York: Morgan Kaufmann.

Xu, Z., S. Jain, and M. Kankanhalli. 2024. "Hallucination Is Inevitable: An Innate Limitation of Large Language Models." *arXiv preprint arXiv:2401.11817*. https://doi.org/10.48550/arXiv.2401.11817

Žižek, S. 1997. *The Plague of Fantasies*. London: Verso.

Žižek, S. 2000. *The Fragile Absolute: Or, Why Is the Christian Legacy Worth Fighting For?* London: Verso.

Žižek, S. 2003. *The Puppet and the Dwarf: The Perverse Core of Christianity*. Cambridge, MA: MIT Press.

Žižek, S. 2006. *The Parallax View*. Cambridge, MA: MIT Press.

Zuboff, S. 2019. *The Age of Surveillance Capitalism: The Fight for a Human Future at the New Frontier of Power*. New York: PublicAffairs.

Zwart, H. 2015. "Extimate Technologies: Empowerment, Intrusiveness, Surveillance: The Fate of the Human Subject in the Age of Intimate Technologies and Big Data." In *Emerging Technologies and Human Rights (Proceedings)*, 40–45. Strasbourg: Council of Europe.

Zwart, H. 2017. "'Extimate' Technologies and Techno-Cultural Discontent: A Lacanian Analysis of Pervasive Gadgets." *Techné: Research in Philosophy and Technology* 21 (1): 24–54.

Zwart, H. 2022. "Psychoanalysis and the Technological Mediation of Subjectivity: A Lacanian Approach." *Journal of Theoretical and Philosophical Psychology* 42 (1): 33–48.

Zwart, H. 2023. "Psychoanalysis and Artificial Intelligence: Discontent, Disruptive Algorithms, and Desire." In L. Possati (Ed.), *Humanizing Artificial Intelligence: Psychoanalysis and the Problem of Control*, 29–49. Berlin: De Gruyter.

Index

Pages in *italics* refer to figures

For Product Safety Concerns and Information please contact our EU representative GPSR@taylorandfrancis.com Taylor & Francis Verlag GmbH, Kaufingerstraße 24, 80331 München, Germany